A WHOLISTIC APPROACH TO EMOTIONAL WELLNESS

I0095807

THE
WAR
FOR
PEACE

SANDRA CASCIATO

THE WAR FOR PEACE:
A Wholistic Approach to Emotional Wellness

Copyright © 2023 by Sandra Casciato

Published by Sandals & Sage
5013 Louise Avenue, Unit #672
Sioux Falls, SD 57108

www.WholisticTransformation.net

Cover design: Doug Newbry
Interior illustrations: iStock (p. 29) and Wikimedia
Interior design: Betty Hopkins
Editorial: April O'Neil
General editor: Betty Hopkins

Paperback book ISBN: 979-8-9872642-0-1
Hardcover book ISBN: 979-8-9872642-1-8
eBook ISBN: 979-8-9872642-2-5

Unless otherwise noted, all Scripture quotations are taken from *BibleGateway.com*,
New King James Version (NKJV).

Health and Medical Disclaimer

This book shares information about the author's personal experiences and opinion about health and wellness. Although great care has been taken to ensure the accuracy of the information presented, the author and the publisher cannot assume responsibility for the validity of all materials or the consequences for their use.

The author is not a medical doctor and is not your healthcare provider. The statements made about products and services have not been evaluated by the U.S. Food and Drug Administration. They are not intended to diagnose, treat, cure, or prevent any condition of disease. Please consult with your personal doctor or medical practitioner regarding the suggestions in this book to determine if they are safe for you.

This book provides information related to physical and mental health issues. Use of this book implies your acceptance of this disclaimer.

This book, *The War for Peace*, is dedicated to my children

Jamin, Nico, and Alexa

You are the bright spot in my life always.

Your unwavering love and support have motivated and inspired me throughout this journey.

I am overwhelmed and humbled that God chose me to be your mother in this earthly realm.

I am grateful that our relationship will continue through eternity.

TABLE OF CONTENTS

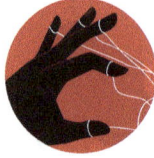

INTRODUCTION

A WHOLISTIC APPROACH TO EMOTIONAL WELLNESS

Every day, you are in a war for the peace and tranquility of your soul. The casualties of this war may not be evident to you or those around you, yet their influence can disrupt every area of your life.

My intention for writing this book is to share some of the myriads of contributors to an imbalanced emotional state and highlight solutions from a wholistic perspective. The categories and examples selected are not exhaustive. They are summaries from personal experience and feedback from people following my protocols. The information presented is confirmed by research and first-hand results. I share this knowledge with the hope that it creates a curiosity in you to challenge the status quo and research the truth for yourself.

This book is a labor of love meant to share my deepest concerns about what we might be missing in our attitudes toward emotional wellness. Unless we take a wholistic approach and consider a variety of possible contributing factors, we may be directing those who are suffering down a single-path solution that can lead to frustration, discouragement, and ongoing suffering.

A Wholistic and Integrative Approach

At the age of 25, when I was first diagnosed with celiac disease*, I weighed 90 pounds and was literally starving to death. After months of pain and testing, I was relieved to learn that through diet and nutrition alone, my body could be restored to health. That was the first time I realized the power of food as medicine. My healing journey led to my study of nutrition, herbalism, and emotional wellness.

As a Vitalist, I encourage root-cause resolutions to illness that consider the physiological, psychological, and spiritual contributors. These contributors are interconnected, and a disconnect in any one of these areas can create an imbalance.

---

* Celiac disease is a reaction to gluten that intercepts the normal absorption of nutrients in the small intestine.

Disintegration

Anxiously, I raced down the hill toward home, leaving the wheels of my Schwinn bike spinning as I dismounted for a quick bathroom stop—not wanting to miss a moment of the fun with the neighborhood regulars. Throwing open the kitchen door of our red brick ranch house, I was immediately paralyzed at the sight in front of me. What I saw and, more importantly, what I believed that day changed me to the core. The 9-year-old who was racing down the hill on her bike and the one standing on the other side of that door was no longer the same person.

As I stood there frozen, I saw my mother's petite body thrashing against my father's angry hands that were gripped around her neck. As her face turned several shades of purple, I knew she was fighting for her life and losing fast. At that moment, the innocent child chose to become a warrior and protector. I would later realize the burden of my decision.

The details that followed are unclear to me, but what I believed at that moment was clear: had I not walked in when I did, I would have lost my mom forever. Surely my hysteria woke my father from his rage, and my mom was safe for the moment. But I never felt safe again and embraced the belief that it was my responsibility to protect my mother at any cost. It

would be 30 years before I fully understood what happened to me that day and how the event unknowingly hijacked my life.

Looking back now as an adult, no one caught in a scenario like this, including myself, would be aware of the impact made in the moment of trauma. After the incident, I rebelled against going to school. Despite my sister's tearful pleas, I refused to board the school bus every morning. Instead, I hiked back up the hill and hid in the backyard until my mother discovered me there. The urge for me to protect her was so overpowering that one day I escaped during recess and walked a mile on a busy highway to get home and make sure my mom was safe. I refused to participate in dance class or Girl Scouts, and leaving the house to play with friends was out of the question. Instead, I played alone on the front porch, or on my swing, or in the treehouse in my backyard. I could not risk my mom being alone if my dad came home from work. I was intensely committed to the assignment. When I was forced to go to school, I was overcome with anxiety until I could be home with my mom again. The shame of what I kept hidden about my family was so isolating that it spiraled me into a state of deep, dark loneliness. The carefree, authentic child in me disappeared.

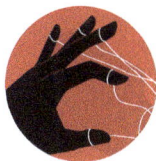

Chapter One

EXTERNAL ASSAULTS TO YOUR MIND

My childhood experiences made me sensitive to those in emotional pain. I was fascinated with understanding human behavior and everything that affects emotions. This curiosity was the catalyst for years of training in psychology, emotional wellness, and natural healing.

This chapter highlights some of the assaults on your physical body that can upset emotional stability. The information is intended to offer awareness so you can take precautionary measures to lessen the negative impact on your body and mind. Personal research is always encouraged.

PHYSIOLOGICAL CONTRIBUTORS

Genetic Predisposition

Historically, scientific consensus held that your physical and psychological health outcomes were at the mercy of your DNA and that this inherited hardwiring could not be changed. In recent decades, however, exciting research in epigenetics shows how external factors can affect the expression of your genes—whether those genes are turned on or off. We now know that your DNA does not have to be your destiny.

Stress and the Allostatic Load

Homeostasis is the process the body uses to maintain a stable set of internal conditions that are necessary for survival. Allostasis is the process of maintaining homeostasis through change and adaptation. [1] The adrenal glands are responsible for producing hormones that will do whatever is necessary to maintain this balance, including modifying set points (blood pressure, breathing, insulin, neurotransmitters).

HOMEOSTASIS and ALLOSTASIS

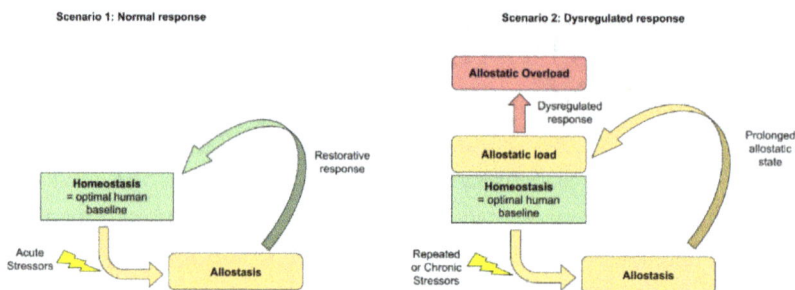

SOURCE: https://www.urbanhealthcouncil.com/

During times of high stress or perceived danger, your body releases cortisol, epinephrine (adrenaline), DHEA, and testosterone to keep you alert and safe. Conversely, thyroid hormones, estrogen, progesterone, growth hormone, and melatonin are decreased. Excess cortisol shrinks your brain, causes cognitive impairment, decreases brain activity, and is associated with Alzheimer's disease. [2]

The combination of stressors—physical, emotional, environmental— and the consequences of continually adapting to chronic stress can create an allostatic load that keeps you in fight-flight-freeze mode. This chronic state can accelerate the risk of disease.

Inflammation

Your immune system is housed mainly in the gut, where inflammatory markers and hormones are passed on to the brain through the vagus nerve. Therefore, the health and stability of the gut have a direct effect on your brain and emotional well-being. Gut inflammation and hormone instability can result from stress, sugar, chemicals, and pathogens, including gluten and GMOs, which can promote intestinal permeability and upset the balance of intestinal flora.

Inflammatory messengers in the blood, called cytokines, are predictive and linearly related to depression and anxiety. Psychiatric researchers have observed that patients with higher levels of inflammatory markers are less likely to respond to antidepressants and more likely to respond to anti-inflammatories. [3, 4]

Isolation

"Solid scientific evidence shows that social relationships affect a range of health outcomes, including mental health, physical health, health habits, and mortality risk." [5] Physical touch is one of the essential contributors to human development and healing. Studies conducted in the 1960s by psychologist Harry Harlow observed the effects of maternal separation and social isolation on the mental and social development of rhesus monkeys. The baby monkeys were separated from their mothers shortly after birth and were nourished by either a surrogate wire mother or a soft, cloth mother. Harlow found that while the monkeys would go to the wire mother for nourishment, they preferred the soft, cloth mother for comfort. The monkeys that only had access to the wire mother would not go to the surrogate for comfort. Instead, when stressed, the baby monkeys threw themselves on the floor and rocked back and forth. Other monkeys were put into an isolation chamber, and within just a few days, the infant monkeys would begin huddling in the corner of the chamber, remaining motionless. Harlow's research resulted in monkeys with severe emotional and social disturbances. They lacked social skills and were unable to play with other monkeys. Harlow's experiments were finally halted in 1985 when the American Psychological Association passed rules regarding the treatment of people and animals in research. [6]

Positive physical touch releases chemicals in the body, such as endorphins, oxytocin (known as the love hormone), and dopamine, which can benefit someone experiencing depression. Alternatively, when touch is invasive, it can create pain and trauma. In some cases, before someone can receive healthy touch, they need to work through the trauma from harmful touch.

Neurotransmitter Imbalance

Neurotransmitters are chemical messengers that transmit signals across a chemical synapse and serve a vital function in your overall emotional health. Therefore, understanding the function, effects, and regulation of these natural chemicals is an essential part of emotional wellness. Later chapters will show how diet, physical activity, and spiritual health positively affect these essential brain chemicals.

Dopamine provides energy, helps control the brain's reward and pleasure centers, and is involved with motivation, novelty, mystery, intelligence, and abstract thought. Dopamine depletion can result in decreased brain power, fatigue, addiction, and loss of attention. [7]

Serotonin calms anxiety and ruminating thoughts. It also helps to maintain deep sleep, a balanced mood, self-confidence, social stability, and a healthy appetite. Low serotonin levels contribute to an overactive prefrontal cortex, depression, anxiety, obsessive-compulsive disorder, aggressive behaviors, suicide, sleep disturbances, eating disorders, emotional volatility, alcohol and drug abuse, and migraines. [8]

Endorphins are feel-good neurotransmitters produced in the brain. There are many ways to boost endorphin levels naturally, such as exercising, laughing with friends, eating chocolate, and engaging in creative activities. The brain also signals the release of endorphins during moments of trauma, stress, fight, flight or freeze, or physical pain to help calm anxiety and relieve pain. Endorphin deficiency can contribute to anxiety, substance abuse, depression, migraines, fibromyalgia, and sleep-wake issues. [9]

GABA contributes to the brain's electrical balance and maintains calm and relaxation. During times of stress or trauma, GABA can be depleted, resulting in bursts of electrical activity called brain arrhythmia. This instability can lead to impulsivity, restlessness, irritability, and the inability to concentrate. [10]

KEY NEUROTRANSMITTERS

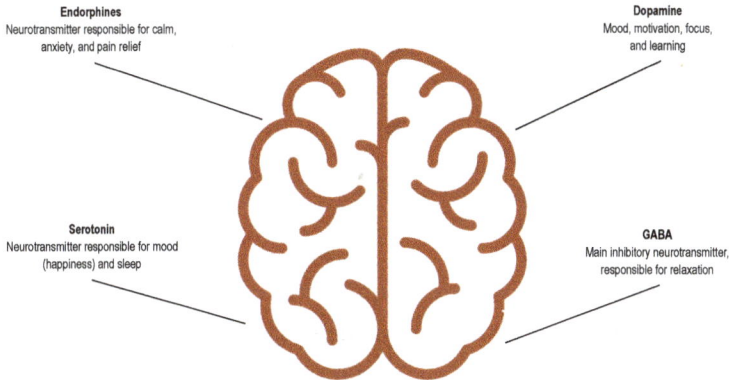

Endorphines
Neurotransmitter responsible for calm, anxiety, and pain relief

Dopamine
Mood, motivation, focus, and learning

Serotonin
Neurotransmitter responsible for mood (happiness) and sleep

GABA
Main inhibitory neurotransmitter, responsible for relaxation

ENVIRONMENTAL CONTRIBUTORS

Every day, you are exposed to harmful chemicals and toxins that can upset your physical, emotional, and mental well-being. Sources include household products, cosmetics, medications, electromagnetic frequencies (EMFs), heavy metals, pesticides, and geoengineering. Previous generations were not exposed to many of these environmental elements that force a heavy burden on your body, requiring ongoing physical adaptation.

In 2005, the Environmental Working Group (EWG) released a report called "Body Burden: The Pollution in Newborns." Researchers at two major laboratories tested umbilical cord blood from 10 babies born in U.S. hospitals between August and September 2004. Tests revealed a total of 287 chemicals in the group, with an average of 200 industrial chemicals and pollutants in each newborn baby (EWG, 2005). [11]

Here are a few of the most common environmental chemicals and their toxic effects.

Pesticides

Multiple studies have shown evidence of pesticide-induced neurodegen-erative and behavioral disorders. Pesticides have shown decreasing glutathione, a powerful antioxidant, while increasing anxiety. Organophosphate pesticides have been shown to act directly on the nervous system by inhibiting the neurotransmitter acetylcholine causing acute psychological and behavioral effects, such as anxiety, depression, and cognitive impairments. [12] The organo-chlorine group of pesticides kills bugs by interfering with GABA receptors, causing them to convulse to death. The GABA system is one of the earliest systems to develop in the fetal brain, and drugs that affect these receptors can cause long-lasting behavioral changes. [13]

Xenoestrogens

Xenoestrogens are synthetic chemicals that mimic estrogen and can accumulate in the body, causing hormone disruption. Estrogen dominance can promote unnatural growth, such as fibroids, cysts, and tumors, as well as weight gain and shifts in mood. Xenoestrogens are used in plastic products in the form of Phthalate and Bisphenol-A (BPA). A leading source of BPA consumption has been through plastic coffee lids. The heat and acidity of the coffee increase the assault of the BPA in the plastic lid. Removing the cover before drinking is an easy solution in this case. These chemicals can also be found in cleaning products, hair products, toothpaste, cosmetics, health and beauty products, shower curtains, flame-retardant clothing, and anything with an artificial scent. Triclosan, a lesser-known xenoestrogen, is used in antibacterial products and sanitizers and has shown a potential risk for cancer. [14]

Mercury

Mercury is considered by toxicologists to be one of the most poisonous naturally occurring substances on the earth. The most common sources of mercury exposure for humans come from dental amalgams, medications, vaccinations, contaminated seafood, mirrors, coal burning, and other indus-trial uses. Symptoms of mercury poisoning include personality changes, insomnia, irritability, impaired concentration, shyness, weakness, apathy, and suicidal disposition. The nervous, immune, and cardiovascular systems suffer the most remarkable effects of chronic mercury exposure. Even low levels of chronic mercury are associated with numerous disorders, including multiple sclerosis, Alzheimer's dementia, Parkinson's disease, and ALS. [15]

From the 1600's to the 1800's, felt hat-makers used quicksilver (mercury nitrate) with disastrous results. A significant number of workers were afflicted with poor memory, inappropriate behavior, shyness, and tremors leading to the "mad hatter" label. Mine workers suffered from crippling neurological and mental disorders after working with Cinnabar, a toxic mercury ore. There are many stories of those affected by mercury toxicity from dental amalgams— from inhaling the vapors to improper removal of fillings containing the metal. Approximately 80% of the mercury released by your fillings is constantly absorbed and stored in your body. Humans get almost seven times more mercury from dental amalgams than from seafood. [16]

IMPORTANT: *If you have mercury fillings that you would like to have removed, consult a biological dentist for proper, safe removal.*

Aluminum

Aluminum can be found in foods, drinking water, aluminum cookware, deodorants, medications, and vaccines. It is highly toxic and has been shown to create damage to the central nervous system. Aluminum can affect cell membranes and myelin sheath surrounding nerve cells, resulting in nerve damage. It also has been found in higher than average amounts in the brains of autistic and Alzheimer's patients. [17] Aluminum builds up in the body over time, hiding in bones, fat, and brain tissue, which makes detoxifying aluminum challenging.

Cooking with acidic foods will cause aluminum pans, baking sheets, or foil to leach aluminum into your food. Stainless steel and glass cookware are better options. Aluminum-based deodorants listed as "antiperspirants" cause aluminum to accumulate in breast tissue and can interfere with estrogen levels. Avoid any deodorant that lists aluminum chloride, aluminum chloro-hydrate, or other aluminum-based ingredients.[18]

Because of aluminum's toxicity, it is often used in vaccines as an "adjuvant" to enhance the body's immune response. As the activated white blood cells are carried into lymph nodes throughout the body and into the brain, they are also delivering the aluminum with them. [19]

Geoengineering / Chemtrails

Geoengineering is the large-scale intervention to alter the Earth's climate with the stated intention of reversing the adverse effects of global warming. Chemtrail spraying involves nano-sized aerosols (aluminum in particular) that are released over the skies and then influenced by electro-magnetic energy to modify the weather. Other aluminum forms do not get absorbed into the body as readily as the aluminum nanoparticles. [20]

When inhaled, these aluminum nanoparticles are absorbed into the brain tissues, where they cause neuro-fibrillary tangles or short circuits in the brain. These short circuits can contribute to neurodegenerative diseases, including Alzheimer's, dementia, Parkinson's disease, and Lou Gehrig's disease (ALS)—all strongly related to exposure to environmental aluminum. Home filtering systems are ineffective at removing the aluminum due to the nano sizing of the aluminum particles being used. [21]

EMFs (Electromagnetic Frequencies)

Electromagnetic frequencies (EMFs) are the radiation emitted by cell phone towers, Wi-Fi, 'smart' utility meters, wireless laptops, baby monitors, cell phones, cordless phones, and other wireless technology. Low levels of natural EMFs can also be found in nature in the form of UV or infrared light, the earth's magnetic field, and other elements. Your body can process a low amount of EMF energy and maintain homeostasis. However, the increasing levels of frequencies from wireless technology place an unprecedented burden on your physical and emotional state, often without your knowledge. The studies on this subject are vast and growing. [22, 23, 24, 25]

In 2013, Dr. Martin Pall at Washington State University discovered the effect of EMFs on calcium channels in the plasma membrane of cells. When EMFs activate these channels, large amounts of intracellular calcium are produced, leading to a chain of chemical reactions resulting in the production of free radicals and oxidative stress. The free radicals then culminate in DNA damage, which can lead to disease. [26]

A 2018 study titled "Thermal and non-thermal health effects of low-intensity non-ionizing radiation" concluded that "there is strong evidence that excessive exposure to mobile phone frequencies over long periods increases the risk of brain cancer both in humans and animals." [27]

Current guidelines for exposure need urgent revision. A study released by the Orebro University Hospital in Sweden by the BioInitiative Working Group 2017 states, "There is a consistent pattern of increased risk for glioma (a malignant brain tumor) and acoustic neuroma with use of mobile and cordless phones." According to Lennart Hardell, MD, Ph.D. "Epidemiological evidence shows that radiofrequency should be classified as a Group 1 (known) human carcinogen." [28, 29]

Epigenetic studies show neurodevelopmental and neurobehavioral changes in young people due to wireless technology resulting in slowed memory, learning, cognition, attention, and behavioral problems. [30]

Sperm exposed to radiofrequency (RF) radiation show decreased motility, morphometric abnormalities, and increased oxidative stress. Men using mobile phones have decreased sperm concentration, decreased motility, and decreased viability.[31,32]

To reduce EMF exposure, use airplane mode on your phone at night or when your phone is near your body. Use the speaker phone when possible, keeping your phone one foot from your body, or use EMF reduction air tube earbuds. Use wired internet instead of wireless in your home, or purchase a router to shut down wireless at night.

LED (Blue Light)

Blue light has a very short wavelength and produces more energy, which is beneficial during daylight hours for boosting attention, reaction times, and mood. The sun is a natural source of blue light. Artificial sources include digital screens, electronic devices, and fluorescent and LED lighting. However, when blue-light exposure is extended artificially, it can disrupt the body's circadian rhythm and restorative processes at night.

Energy-saving, light-emitting diode (LED) lights release blue light that can generate high amounts of oxidative stress. Medical evidence shows that blue light exposure may cause permanent eye damage and contribute to age-related macular degeneration, which can lead to vision loss.

Exposure to blue light also affects your ability to produce enough melatonin to achieve quality sleep. A lack of melatonin increases your risk for mood disorders, heart disease, stroke, and obesity. Melatonin has anti-inflammatory and antitumor effects and is involved in aging and longevity. The most critical functions of melatonin are autophagy (cleaning out the dysfunctional components of a cell) and apoptosis (programmed cell death), which guard against cancer and major neurocognitive disorders, such as dementia. [33, 34, 35, 36, 37]

Here are some simple ways to counteract the negative effects of blue light:

- Use dim red lights for night lights
- Avoid looking at bright screens two to three hours before bed
- Use blue-light-blocking glasses while using electronic devices
- Install an app that filters the blue/green wavelength at night
- Use lighting with safer ratings, such as incandescent
- Use melatonin to balance your circadian rhythm
- Eat foods high in omega-3 fats and anthocyanins to protect your sight

Toxic Mold

While most molds you encounter daily are not dangerous, some produce gas-like substances called mycotoxins. Mycotoxins pose a severe threat to human health when inhaled, swallowed, or absorbed through the skin. Though very prevalent, toxic mold illness is routinely undiagnosed. [38, 39]

Mold allergies, which cause symptoms similar to hay fever, are not the same as mold toxicity. Toxic mold results from the volatile toxic vapors produced by mold that can cause a chronic inflammatory response (CIRS), an auto-immune reaction caused by poor clearance of biotoxins in vulnerable individuals. Approximately 25% of the population has an immune response gene called HLA-DR that inhibits the clearing of these mycotoxins from their body, making them more susceptible to the effects of mold exposure. [40]

Mold growth is initiated through water damage and can grow on damp walls, wallpaper, floor and carpet dust, humidifiers, HVAC fans, and stored food products. Mycotoxin production comes from many types of mold, the most common being Stachybotrys Chartarum, also called "black mold," which is the most toxic. Other common toxic molds include Aspergillus flavus, which can form aflatoxins, a known carcinogen.

Fumigatus fungus is one of the most prevalent airborne molds which produces gliotoxin, which can inhibit the communication pathways between immune cells. Aspergillus Versicolor is associated with pulmonary disease.[41]

Mycotoxin exposure can manifest in a variety of ways. Here are some symptoms of concern, particularly those that affect brain and emotional health:

COGNITIVE IMPAIRMENT. Brain fog and memory loss.

DEPRESSION AND ANXIETY. A study of over 5,000 adults published in the American Journal of Public Health found that those living in moldy environments had significantly higher rates of depression compared to those living in mold-free environments. [42]

NEUROLOGIC AND NEUROPSYCHIATRIC SYNDROME. "Human exposure to molds, mycotoxins, and water-damaged buildings can cause neurologic and neuropsychiatric signs and symptoms. Many of these clinical features can partly mimic or be similar to classic neurologic disorders, including pain syndromes, movement disorders, delirium, dementia, and disorders of balance and coordination." [43]

ADDITIONAL SYMPTOMS. Headaches, insomnia, chronic fatigue, leaky gut, autoimmune disease, food sensitivities, histamine intolerance, fibromyalgia, joint and muscle pain, light sensitivity, blurred vision, skin sensitivity, mood swings, confusion, disorientation, sinus problems, shortness of breath, and Lyme disease symptoms (though testing negative for Lyme disease). [44, 45, 46]

If you think you may have been exposed to toxic mold, hire a mold specialist to analyze your home and treat any mold problem immediately. Find a health practitioner that specializes in mycotoxin recovery with a successful track record in treating mold toxicity. The International Society for Environmentally Acquired Illness specializes in environmentally acquired illness (EAI) and provides resources, including education and referrals to medical professionals. [47]

PHARMACEUTICAL CONTRIBUTORS

When it comes to your physical and mental health, you need to be your own advocate. That starts with information backed by scientific research, with all possible options considered so that you can make an informed decision for your long-term health and well-being. Of primary importance is an understanding of what is happening physiologically and psychologically that may have contributed to your current state of health.

The four categories of medications reviewed in this section are some of the most commonly prescribed drugs that may negatively impact emotional health.

IMPORTANT DISCLAIMER: *I am not a medical professional and recommend that you check with your doctor before withdrawing from any medications you are taking. It is also wise to check with your doctor before starting any new medications or supplements. It can be extremely dangerous to halt medications abruptly, and it is important that you make any transitions with the guidance of a medical physician. The information presented here is from my research and experience and is shared for educational purposes only. I urge you to advocate for your own health, which involves doing your own research.*

Statin Drugs

A quarter of all the cholesterol in your body is found in your brain and plays a crucial role in brain signaling and neuron growth. Statin drugs suppress the synthesis of cholesterol, deplete your brain of coenzyme Q10 (CoQ10) and neurotransmitter precursors, and interfere with the delivery of essential fatty acids and fat-soluble antioxidants to your brain. Research shows that the best memory function in older adults was observed in those with the highest levels of cholesterol. [48, 49] Conversely, low cholesterol is associated with an increased risk of depression and even death. [50] In a study from the University of California, San Diego, 90 percent of patients reported improvement in cognitive problem solving within a couple of weeks after discontinuing statin medication. Some patients experienced a reversal of the diagnosis of dementia or Alzheimer's disease.[51]

Antidepressants / SSRIs

In six decades, not one study has proven that a chemical imbalance in the brain causes depression. There is no standardized medical test to measure brain chemical levels that cause depression. Therefore, no prescription can restore to a normal state that is undefined. Even when these psychoactive substances provide relief, they are not correcting an under-lying chemical imbalance in the brain and can potentially create neurological imbalances that were not there previously. Functional Psychiatrist Kelly Brogan formerly supported anti-depressant treatment with her patients until finding evidence that they resulted in worse long-term outcomes. They are debilitatingly habit-forming, and their use may permanently disable the body's self-healing potential. According to Dr. Brogan, the best way to heal the mind is to heal the whole body. [52]

In her TED Talk, "Why We Love, Why We Cheat," Dr. Helen Fisher explains that SSRIs raise serotonin while suppressing dopamine and the resulting oxytocin and vasopressin that are associated with romantic love and attachment.[53]

Researchers in a 2009 study of 14,000 depressed patients concluded that there was no link between low serotonin and depression, nor any link between stressful life events and changes to serotonin levels. Rather, it was the number of stressful life events that were significantly associated with depression. [54]

In a 2015 study titled "Is Serotonin an Upper or a Downer?" researchers expressed concern over selective serotonin reuptake inhibitors (SSRIs), which artificially elevate the brain's serotonin levels. Their research shows that high serotonin levels, not low serotonin, have been linked to multiple depressive disorders. When SSRIs artificially elevate serotonin, energy homeostasis is disrupted, and symptoms can become worse.[55]

In a September 2018 paper published in BMJ Evidence-Based Medicine, Michael P. Hengartner, a clinical psychologist at the Zurich University of Applied Sciences, concludes that there is no evidence that antidepressants are clinically effective for any form of depression—whether mild, moderate, or severe. Any effect indicated is incredibly small, only slightly more than that of a placebo, and is not clinically meaningful. Another study published by Hengartner, with Jules Angst and Wulf Rossler, found that after 30 years, people who took antidepressants had worsening symptoms over time. [56]

A 2018 qualitative study published in the British Journal of Psychiatry reported adverse emotional side effects of SSRIs, which participants strongly attributed to their antidepressant medication. Although negative emotions reduced at some stage, many felt that the emotional side effects hindered their quality of life. These adverse effects included headache, increased anxiety, agitation, blunting of emotions, as well as changes in sleep, gastrointestinal and sexual functioning. A few participants did not experience any emotions, while others experienced emotions as "cognitive" or "intellectual" thoughts rather than as feelings. Most participants described feeling emotionally detached, more like a spectator than a participant. Almost all participants described a reduction in their positive emotions, including happiness, enjoyment, excitement, anticipation, passion, love, affection, and enthusiasm. Some participants described similarities between the SSRI-induced state and depression itself and suggested that the medication might increase or induce a kind of depression." [57]

It is important to research and understand all available options so you can make an informed decision on the best treatment for you. Then, work with your doctor to start with safer alternatives when possible.

WARNING: *Decreasing or stopping medications can be very dangerous. Withdrawal symptoms are often used as confirmation that the medication is needed when the symptoms are the result of your body withdrawing from the medication. If you are in a life-threatening situation, seek immediate professional help. Always work with your medical doctor to make any modifications to your prescription intake.*

Benzodiazepines

Alprazolam is the most commonly prescribed psychotropic medication in the United States. It belongs to a group of drugs called benzodiazepines (aka benzos) which are used to treat anxiety and panic disorders by increasing the production of the calming chemical GABA. However, the body eventually builds up a tolerance to them, and more of the medication is needed to feel the original effects. According to a study in the Journal of Addictive Medicine, "Long-term use of benzodiazepine, in general, is controversial and not recommended, although commonly practiced. Interestingly, tolerance was found to develop relatively quickly for the hypnotic, sedative, and anticonvulsant actions of all benzodiazepines." [58]

Common adverse effects include drowsiness, insomnia, memory impairment, anxiety, irritability, headache, nausea, decreased libido, worsening depression, hypomania, and decreased mental alertness. [59, 60]

In her book *Drug Muggers*, pharmacist Susie Cohen explains how anti-anxiety medication depletes melatonin, which can lead to more anxiety, and how niacin (B3) works as a natural, milder tranquilizer. Studies show its effect is similar to benzo medications and has been used by doctors in Italy to wean patients from benzo medications.[61]

Additional information is available at *BenzoBuddies.org*, a benzodiazepine withdrawal support group.

CAUTION: *Consult your doctor before stopping or decreasing any medications to avoid serious side effects. If you want to taper from benzodiazepines, it is critical that you do so very slowly and with the assistance of your doctor.*

Fluoroquinolone Antibiotics

Fluoroquinolones are one of the most commonly prescribed antibiotics in the United States, and they can lead to chronic illness and permanent disability with no known cure. These broad-spectrum antibiotics work like chemotherapy agents, disrupting DNA and destroying cells. The fluorinated quinolones administer the potent neurotoxin fluoride directly into the body's tissues. Fluoroquinolones are known to cause mitochondrial damage and oxidative stress, which can lead to a host of illnesses ranging from minor disturbances to complete debilitation. Reactions may be immediate or delayed, even years after stopping the antibiotic.

Fluoroquinolone-associated disability (FQAD) can last for years and may include damage to the peripheral nervous system, central nervous system, musculoskeletal system, cardiovascular system, gastrointestinal system, skin, and senses. Symptoms include insomnia, anxiety, depression, fatigue, memory impairment, and personality changes. [62, 63, 64, 65]

In July 2016, the U.S. Food and Drug Administration approved safety labeling changes for fluoroquinolones to enhance warnings about their association with disabling and potentially permanent side effects and to limit their use in patients with less serious bacterial infections.[66]

My Experience with Fluoroquinolone Toxicity

I learned about fluoroquinolone toxicity the hard way when I was prescribed the medication for a minor infection. I rarely use medications, but since I was heading out of town for two weeks, I opted for what I thought would be a quick fix. Unfortunately, shortly after completing the medication, I became physically ill with flu-like symptoms and spent three days in bed. After returning home, I started to feel very melancholy and gradually spiraled downward into depression and despair. For over a week, I was weepy and felt completely hopeless for no known reason. I had never struggled with depression, so this was terrifying to me. I did a deep herbal cleanse with lots of distilled water, and within a few days, the cleansing released the circulating toxins from my body, and immediately, my state of mind shifted back to normal. I was amazed and relieved.

It wasn't until months later that I learned what triggered the erratic symptoms that I had experienced. I attended a seminar where countless stories were shared by those who had been "floxed" and the resulting physical and mental symptoms they endured from fluoroquinolone antibiotics, some lasting for years. [67] I am grateful for the knowledge I gained from my experience and that I can share it to bring awareness to others.

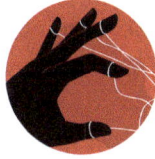

Chapter Two

FOOD AND MOOD

*Let food be thy medicine, and
medicine be thy food.*

— Hippocrates

What you eat can affect your emotions, and your emotions can affect what you eat. Your gut and brain are in constant communication via the vagus nerve that connects your gastrointestinal tract with your central nervous system. This bio-signaling is known as the gut-brain axis. It is estimated that 95% of the body's serotonin is produced in the gut. Research has shown that depression, anxiety, and several mood disorders have been correlated to alterations in serotonergic pathways. [1, 2, 3]

Maintaining optimal health in your gastrointestinal tract is essential when addressing your mental state. Factors that adversely affect the gut microbiome include inflammation, chronic stress, chemicals, drugs, and foods such as sugar, refined carbohydrates, and gluten.

The Culprits

Gluten

The relationship of celiac disease to neurologic and psychiatric complications has been observed for over 40 years. Many studies support the gluten-mood connection in anxiety, social phobia, depression, and schizophrenia. Removing gluten from the diet often results in the reversal of psychiatric and neurological symptoms. Gluten can compromise the blood-brain barrier as well as the tight junctions in the intestinal lining, making each more permeable—a term referred to as leaky brain and leaky gut. When proteins escape from the gut into the bloodstream, they can create inflammation and autoimmunity. [4, 5]

Glyphosate and GMOs

Glyphosate is the most widely used herbicide on food crops in the world, with nearly one billion pounds applied every year. It has been shown to cause nutritional deficiencies, especially minerals (which are critical for brain function and mood control) and systemic toxicity. Dr. Stephanie Seneff's study on the effects of glyphosate (the active ingredient in Roundup® weed killer, used on nearly all GMO crops) found that "glyphosate's adverse effects on the gut microbiota can remarkably explain a great number of the diseases and conditions that are prevalent in the modern industrialized world." [6, 7]

Vegetable Oils

A high intake of N6 vegetable fats—corn, safflower, sunflower, peanut, canola, and soybean oils—has been shown to impair brain function and to increase the risk of neurodegenerative diseases as well as cancer, diabetes, atherosclerosis, heart attacks, and strokes. It's estimated that we consume 50 times more N-6 fats than necessary for good health. [8]

Refined Carbohydrates

Foods high in refined carbohydrates cause your insulin to spike, which leads to inflammation, and unmanaged inflammation leads to disease. [9]

Limiting carbohydrate intake and choosing complex carbohydrates that contain fiber to regulate the rise of insulin can help to regulate weight and mood. Diabetics (type 1 or type 2) have an increased risk of developing depression. [10]

Monosodium Glutamate (MSG)

MSG is routinely added to processed low-quality foods to artificially enhance the flavor. High levels of glutamate in the blood can bypass the protective blood-brain barrier causing brain cells to shrivel and die. Even in lower concentrations, glutamate can damage neural connections called synapses. The greatest damage in Alzheimer's disease is not the cell bodies but the synaptic connections. Therefore, even low exposure to MSG should be avoided. [11]

Sugar

Sugar feeds pathogens in your gut, which destroy beneficial bacteria. It depletes B vitamins, zinc, and magnesium and can cause fatigue, moodiness, nervousness, and depression. Sugar suppresses the production of a key growth hormone called brain-derived neurotrophic factor (BDNF), which plays an important role in reducing anxiety, panic, and stress. Long-term, sugar can contribute to the shrinking of your hippocampus, which is involved with the formation, organization, and storage of memories. [12, 13, 14]

The glycemic index (GI) is a valuable tool to measure how carbohydrates affect blood glucose levels. Foods are classified on a scale of 0–100 as low (55 or less), medium (56–69), or high (70+) glycemic foods. The lower the GI ranking of a specific food, the less it may affect your blood sugar level. The glycemic load (GL) is a measurement that accounts for the quantity and quality of the carbohydrate content and its resulting effect on blood glucose levels. The formula to calculate glycemic load is: GL = GI × carbohydrate / 100. Foods with a glycemic load of 10g or less are low, 11–19g are medium, and 20g or more are high. [15, 16]

Aspartame

The artificial sweetener aspartame contains methanol which is converted in the body to formaldehyde (a known carcinogen, used as a preservative and former embalming fluid) and formic acid (a poison used by the fire ant which causes intense pain). "There is evidence that aspartame can worsen depression in those already suffering from the condition, may cause weight gain and insomnia, worsen diabetic control, aggravate multiple sclerosis and other neurological diseases, trigger migraine headaches and seizures, cause blindness, and may also damage a fetus' developing brain." [17]

A study published in the Journal of Toxicology and Environmental Health Part A, sites "evidence that, in the animals studied, Splenda reduces the number of good bacteria in the intestines by 50%, increases the pH level in the intestines, and contributes to increases in body weight." [18]

General Dietary Recommendations

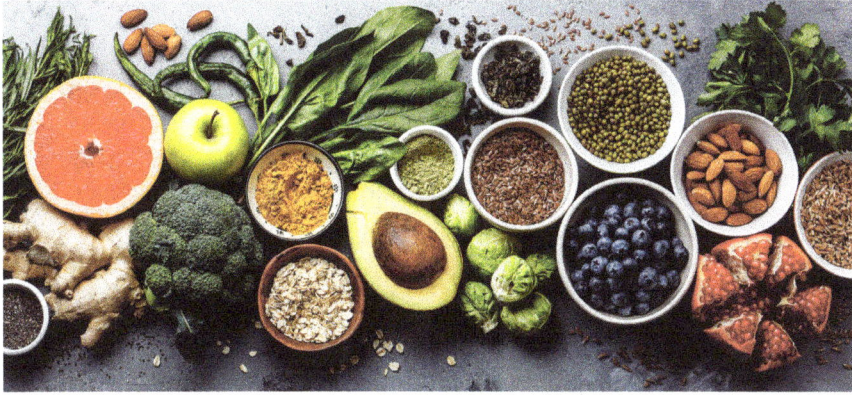

The following food recommendations are for people who are in general good health with no dietary restrictions. Choose organic, non-GMO foods with minimal processing to support brain health and positive mood. Avoid canned, packaged, and processed foods with unnecessary and potentially harmful ingredients.

Greens and Vegetables. Selecting raw or cooked vegetables in assorted colors (for a variety of antioxidants) is a foundational part of any healthy diet. Cruciferous vegetables like broccoli, cabbage, cauliflower, Brussels sprouts, arugula, watercress, radish, and kale are rich in fiber, minerals, and antioxidants with anti-inflammatory and anti-cancer properties.

Protein. A great source of energy that balances blood sugar levels and keeps your mood steady is protein. The best protein options include organic-pastured-raised chicken and eggs, wild-caught fish, and grass-fed beef.

Omega-3 Fats. These fats (EPH and DHA), predominately found in fish, promote healthy brain function and enhance emotional well-being. Wild-caught fish is preferred as it is more nutritionally dense than farmed fish. Smaller fish have less mercury and are the best choice. The Environmental Working Group (EWG) recommends the following fish that are very high in omega-3s, low in mercury, and sustainable: wild salmon, sardines, mussels, rainbow trout, and Atlantic mackerel. Avoid fish high in mercury, such as: king mackerel, marlin, orange roughy, bluefin, bigeye tuna, shark, swordfish, and tilefish. [19]

Healthy Fats. Approximately 60% of your brain is composed of fat. Several studies found that low intakes of DHA-type fats increase the likelihood of depression and that restoring DHA can relieve it. Healthy fats include avocado, coconut oil, grass-fed butter, ghee (clarified butter), and olive oil. Extra virgin olive oil contains a high amount of oleic acid, which researchers have shown to have powerful anti-cancer effects, along with flavonoids that prevent inflammation and neutralize free radicals. Grass-fed butter, ghee, and coconut oil are best for cooking at high heat.

Nuts and Seeds. These are a great source of healthy fats and make a satisfying snack. Raw and unsalted is best, as roasting can create free radicals, which can damage your cells. The best choices are pecans, walnuts, almonds, macadamia nuts, Brazil nuts, sunflower seeds, pumpkin seeds, chia seeds, and flaxseeds. Nut butters should be unsweetened and preferably organic and raw.

Complex Carbohydrates. Always in moderation, complex carbohydrates are a nutritious option to replace refined carbohydrates. They include whole grains, legumes, fruit, seeds, nuts, quinoa, sweet potatoes, and brown rice.

Low-Glycemic Fruits. Berries are a great choice as they are high in antioxidants and lower in sugar content. Fruits with a higher glycemic index (GI) should be eaten in moderation.

Fermented Foods. Kimchi, sauerkraut, yogurt, kefir, miso, and tempeh are rich sources of nutrients and phytochemicals with anti-microbial and anti-carcinogenic properties. The prebiotic and probiotic properties of fermented foods contribute to healthy gut microbiota composition. The antioxidant properties neutralize free radicals, reduce oxidative stress, improve inflammatory responses, and enhance the immune system. [20, 21]

Sweeteners. Whole foods such as honey, maple syrup, and molasses are healthier options for sweeteners when used in moderation. They provide vitamins, minerals, and antioxidants which support your immune system. Unlike refined sugars, they do not produce an insulin spike followed by a crash in blood sugar. Instead, they provide a slow, even rise of insulin with a slow energy burn. [22, 23] Natural, sugar-free options include stevia and monk fruit. Caution is advised when using sugar alcohols, such as Erythritol and Xylitol, as they can cause gastrointestinal upset and headache.

Beverages. Drinking pure water is essential for removing toxins from your body. An average of half your body weight in ounces is recommended daily. My preference is steam-distilled water which is H_2O only and provides the additional benefit of attracting and removing inorganic minerals from the body. Reverse osmosis is another good option. Avoid fluoridated water. [24]

Theanine, found in green and black tea, promotes mental clarity and produces a calming effect on the brain. Studies show that L-theanine reduces psychological and physiological stress responses and increases serotonin, dopamine, and GABA levels. One study showed that L-theanine reduces anxiety in patients with schizophrenia when added to antipsychotic therapy.[25, 26] Studies suggest that tea drinking is associated with lower risks of cognitive impairment and decline, and found that the protective effect was not limited to a particular type of tea. [27, 28]

Herbal teas provide many health benefits and come in various flavors. Specific herbs for emotional wellness are discussed in detail in Chapter Four.

Coffee (1 to 2 cups a day) can contribute to a general sense of well-being. It triggers the release of BDNF, which has an antidepressant effect and improves brain health. [29]

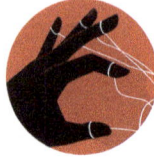

Chapter Three

NUTRIENTS TO ENHANCE BRAIN AND MOOD

Over the last 40 years, nutrient levels in our foods have been significantly depleted. Agricultural practices have contributed to this loss with mass farming, the use of pesticides and herbicides, near elimination of crop rotation, and failure to allow the land to rest and replenish. High-temperature cooking further destroys vitamins, minerals, and antioxidants in the food. Taking a daily vitamin and mineral supplement is more important today than it was for our grandparents. Whole food supplements are preferred as they are recognized by the body and have a better chance of proper assimilation. Supplements specific for brain and emotional health include:

Omega-3 fatty acids, eicosatetraenoic acid (EPA), and docosahexaenoic acid (DHA) are among the fats that make up nearly 60 percent of our brains. These omega-3 fatty acids are critical for supporting brain function and mood, regulating metabolism, and preventing diabetes and inflammation. Low blood levels of omega-3s are associated with brain shrinkage, memory loss, and cognitive function decline.[1]

Probiotics are beneficial bacteria that nourish and protect the gut/brain communication pathways. Without the right diversity of gut bacteria, inflammation and leaky brain can occur, which can contribute to brain fog and dementia.

Magnesium is one of the most essential minerals involved in protecting the brain, and depletion of this critical mineral has been shown in the hippocampus of those with Alzheimer's disease.[2] Research shows that about 75 percent of people are deficient in magnesium, which plays an important role in more than 300 enzymatic reactions in the body.

Vitamin D provides anti-inflammatory and immune-boosting properties necessary for brain health and cognitive function. Unfortunately, more than 80 percent of the American population has insufficient vitamin D levels, which can contribute to a wide range of problems, including dementia. Researchers believe optimal vitamin D levels may enhance the amount of important chemicals in your brain that assist in bringing damaged neurons back to health.

CoQ10 increases cellular glutathione levels and has been shown to improve memory and other brain functions.[3]

Vitamins C and E protect brain cells from oxidative damage and protect microvessels that feed the brain. Studies have shown that vitamin C supplementation seems to protect the brain against Alzheimer's disease and age-related memory loss.[4]

B vitamins are involved with good brain health and protection from degeneration. Thiamine and riboflavin are involved in energy production, and folic acid, B12, B6, and niacinamide all contribute to DNA repair and synthesis. B6 is involved in the production of neurotransmitters, including serotonin and dopamine. B12 protects the brain and nervous system, regulates rest and mood cycles, and keeps the immune system functioning properly. A severe B12 deficiency can lead to deep depression, paranoia and delusions, difficulty thinking and reasoning, and memory loss.[5]

Alpha-lipoic acid (ALA) is a powerful antioxidant, energy generator, and metal chelator (of arsenic, cadmium, and mercury) that protects the liver and encourages the regeneration of damaged liver cells. It also significantly enhances cellular glutathione levels.[6]

Acetyl-L-carnitine (ALC) increases mitochondrial energy formation, chelates iron, increases brain glutathione levels and increases brain levels of CoQ10. Studies have shown acetyl-L-carnitine's ability to significantly slow and even reverse the effects of aging on the brain.[7]

N-acetyl cysteine (NAC) is essential for the body to replenish glutathione, a powerful antioxidant that plays a vital role in your body's detoxification process. NAC has been shown to alleviate symptoms for those with depression, OCD, and schizophrenia.[8, 9, 10]

NOTE: *The U.S. Food & Drug Association (FDA) has not evaluated these statements. This information is not intended to diagnose, treat, cure, or prevent any disease. Always consult with your doctor before combining supplements with any medications you are taking.*

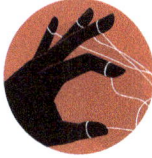

Chapter Four

HERBS FOR EMOTIONAL SUPPORT

NOTE: *The information shared here is for educational purposes only and is based on the historical and traditional use of herbs in maintaining and promoting good health. It is not intended for diagnosing any disease or prescribing any treatment. This information has not been evaluated by the FDA. Consult with your doctor if you are under medical care or taking prescription medication before adding any herbal supplements to your diet. Not recommended for pregnant or nursing mothers or children.*

Herbal medicine is the oldest form of therapy practiced by humankind. There are no people known to anthropology, however isolated or primitive, who did not practice some form of plant medicine. Almost every tribe has its medicine man or woman, who is the living repository of medical knowledge.[1] Herbs have co-existed with man since the beginning of recorded history and are therefore recognized and assimilated by your body more easily than processed and refined foods or chemical medicines. The alkaline nature of plants helps stabilize your body's pH levels which supports your body's healing processes. Unlike medicines, herbs cannot be patented since they are created by God, and therefore, limited funds are invested in research because there is little profit to be made.

Herbs and herbal products are not all medicinally equal. When purchasing herbs, the integrity of the farm or manufacturer is of primary consideration to ensure the highest quality product, free of GMOs, pesticides, and herbicides. Although herbs are natural, that does not ensure safety. Some plants can be dangerous to ingest or even touch. Extreme caution is advised when foraging herbs in the wild unless you are well-educated in plant identification.

Essential Oils (EOs), compounds extracted from plants through distillation, are commonly used for aromatherapy, applied to the skin using a carrier oil, or for scenting body creams, candles, and cleaning products—a superior option to toxic perfumes and chemical scents. Unlike whole herb extracts, essential oils can require several pounds of a plant to create one bottle and do not include the supportive constituents of that plant. The result is a product that is far more potent and, therefore, not recommended for internal consumption. Use essential oils wisely, purchase from a reputable source, and read the label, as many essential oil products include other ingredients, including chemicals. Look for those stating 100% essential oil with no other fillers. When used internally, whole herbs are best—freshly cut, dried, in capsules, or as a liquid extract.

Cleanse • Nourish • Heal

Removing toxins from the body is extremely beneficial to emotional wellness. Toxins can recirculate throughout your body if they are unable to be eliminated because of blockages in the elimination pathways. There is a specific order to detox for the best results: lower bowel, kidneys, liver, and then the bloodstream. The lower bowel must be cleansed first to be able to receive and process toxins from the other organs. Any stagnation in the liver and kidneys will cause toxins from the bloodstream to back up.

The herbs listed in this chapter are those that I have personally used for over ten years. Consideration should be given to the biological uniqueness of each person and how their system utilizes or reacts to any food or supplement. The guidance of a trained herbalist is recommended when incorporating any new herbal therapy. If you have any medical conditions or if you are taking prescription medications, check with your doctor before adding herbs to your diet. None of the herbs listed are recommended for pregnant women, nursing mothers, or children.

Brain and Central Nervous System Herbs

The herbs in this section stimulate circulation, deliver oxygen to the brain to assist with mental alertness, nourish the central nervous system to calm and/ or stimulate according to the body's needs, and balance mood.

Ginkgo (Ginkgo biloba) is one of the oldest living tree species and has been used in China for thousands of years for various ailments. Ginkgo is high in magnesium, phosphorus, potassium, and quercetin. It has been shown to significantly increase oxygen and blood flow in all organs and tissues, including the brain and heart muscles. Ginkgo protects brain cells in the hippocampus from beta-amyloid injury (toxic plaque seen in the brains of Alzheimer's patients) and is protective of the brain's neuron synapses. [2] Some reported benefits include improved memory, concentration, mental alertness, and a sense of physical and emotional well-being. [3, 4]

In a study of Alzheimer's patients given Ginkgo biloba extract, improvement was observed in the group of patients with very mild to mild cognitive impairment, while in more severe dementia, ginkgo functioned more to stabilize or slow down the worsening of the condition. [5]

The Commission E*, considered the world's foremost authority on herbal therapies, has licensed Ginkgo in Germany for the treatment of cerebral dysfunction, including memory deficits, disturbances in concentration, and depressive emotional condition. [6]

CAUTION: *Consult your doctor if taking blood thinning medication, as Ginkgo biloba has a mild blood thinning effect. Avoid using with MAO inhibitors.*

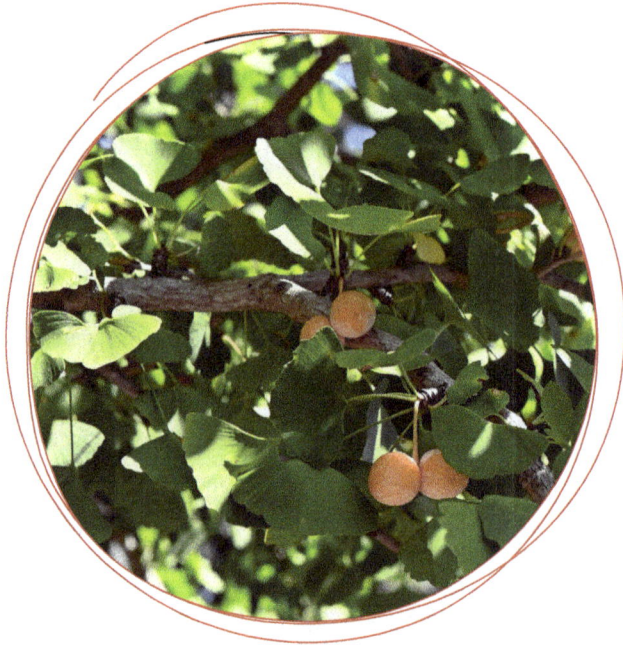

SOURCE: Wikimedia. Ginkgo biloba fruit on a branch.

Rosemary (Rosmarinus officinalis) has a long-lived reputation for improving memory and has been traditionally known as the remembrance herb. It is an analgesic, antidepressant, anti-inflammatory, antioxidant, and encephalic. It improves circulation, increases mental activity, focus, and concentration, supports the function of the liver, and helps to lower blood sugar.

---

 * The Commission E is an expert panel of physicians and scientists having expertise in herbal medicine and related disciplines. In 1978 the Commission was formed as a division of the German Federal Health Agency to evaluate the safety and efficacy of over 300 herbal medicines sold in German pharmacies.

A key element of rosemary is 1,8-cineole, which can enter the blood-stream by inhalation, cross the blood-brain barrier, and inhibit the enzymes that break down acetylcholine, the principal neurotransmitter in the brain, which helps synapses fire. Additionally, 1,8-cineole increases dopamine release in brain cells. [7, 8, 9, 10]

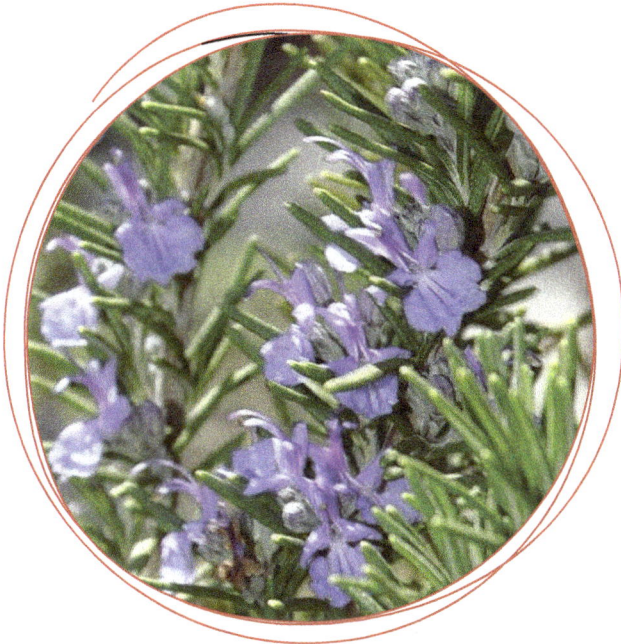

SOURCE: Wikimedia. Rosemary (Rosmarinus officinalis).
Photo by David J. Stang

Valerian Root (Valeriana officinalis) is a nervine, sedative, and antispas-modic. For thousands of years, the Chinese, Greeks, Romans, and Indians have used valerian as a mild sedative. Its therapeutic uses were described by Hippocrates and in the second century, Galen prescribed valerian for insomnia. In the sixteenth century, it was used to treat nervousness, trembling, headaches, and heart palpitations. [11, 12, 13] Valerian is high in calcium, iron, and riboflavin (B2). It also contains ascorbic acid, beta-carotene, selenium, magnesium, potassium, quercetin, and zinc. In a controlled, double-blind clinical trial, valerian root in combination with St. John's wort was reported to be more effective than Valium. [14]

CAUTION: *Consult your doctor before taking valerian if you are taking sedating prescription medications. Do not use in depressive states unless combined with stimulating herbs.*

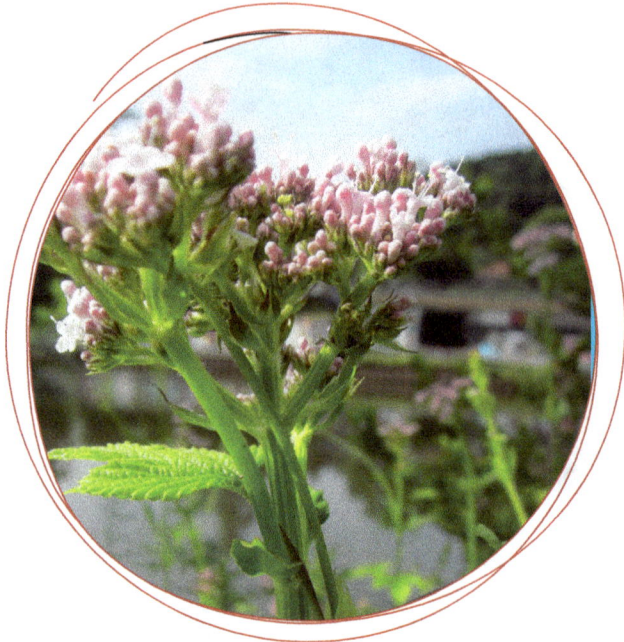

SOURCE: Wikimedia. Valerian Root (Valeriana Officinalis).

Skullcap (Scutellaria lateriflora) is a nervine, anti-spasmodic, anticonvulsant, parasympathetic (rest and digest) herb that tones and soothes the nervous system. It has been beneficial for raw nerves, epilepsy, and motor nerve injury. The herb's active phytochemical compounds contribute to the anxiolytic (anti-anxiety) effects by binding to the benzodiazepine site of the GABA-A receptor. The British Herbal Compendium recognizes the use of skullcap for headaches, migraines, panic attacks, and sleep disorders as well as restlessness and nervous disorders due to anxiety, tension, and stress. Skullcap also can assist with the withdrawal from benzodiazepines. [15] Skullcap is high in magnesium and contains calcium, Vitamin C, iron, B vitamins, zinc, and quercetin.

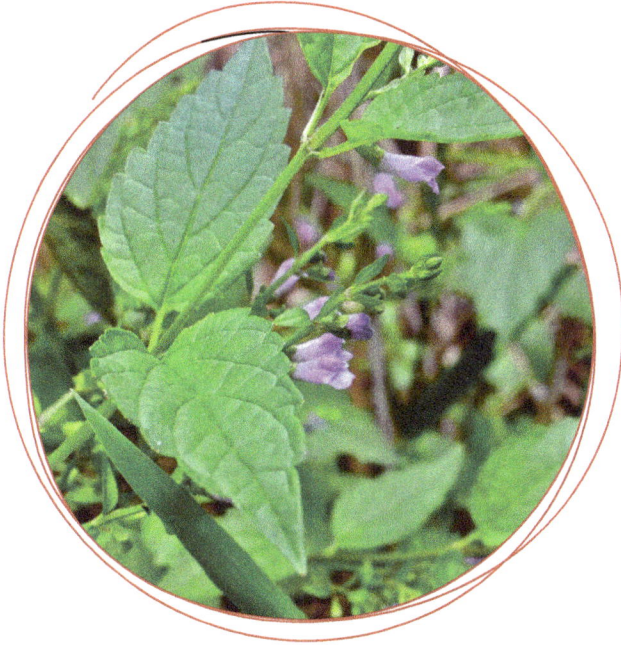

SOURCE: Wikimedia. Scutellaria lateriflora—Blue Skullcap.
Photo by Fritz Flohr Reynolds.

Black Cohosh (Cimicifuga racemosa) regulates and normalizes hormone production and is highly regarded as a nervine and muscle relaxant as it feeds, regulates, strengthens, and rebuilds the nervous system. Black Cohosh contains trace amounts of most known vitamins. With anti-spasmodic, astringent, nervine, and sedative properties, it has been used for epilepsy, nervous excitability, tremors, neuralgia, hysteria, and nerve inflammation. [16]

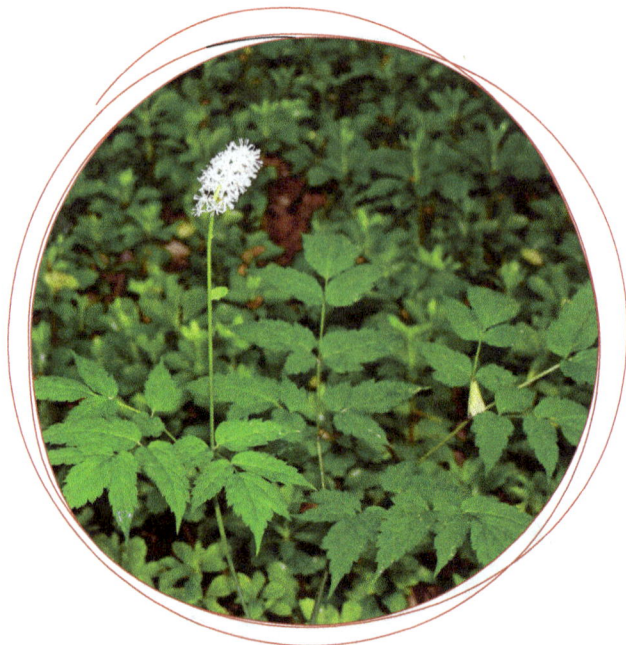

SOURCE: Wikimedia. Black Cohosh (Cimicifuga racemosa).
Photo by SB Johnny.

St. John's Wort (Hypericum perforatum) has been proven in scientific studies to mimic the effects of antidepressant drugs by inhibiting the breakdown of three of the four known feel-good neurotransmitters, serotonin, norepinephrine, and dopamine. It is prescribed throughout the world as a mild antidepressant that can elevate mood, stimulate the nerves, and strengthen immunity. As a nervine stimulant, St. John's Wort (SJW) has been helpful in treating neuralgia, depression, anxiety, and sleep disturbances. It has antiviral, antibacterial, and anti-inflammatory qualities and aids with liver detoxification. [17,]

CAUTION: *It is not recommended to combine SJW with antidepressant drugs. St. John's Wort may reduce the effectiveness of oral contraceptives, and high doses may lead to photosensitivity. Do not take with protease inhibitors (used for HIV/ AIDS) or cyclosporine. Consult your doctor before combining SJW with any medication or discontinuing medication for depression or anxiety.*

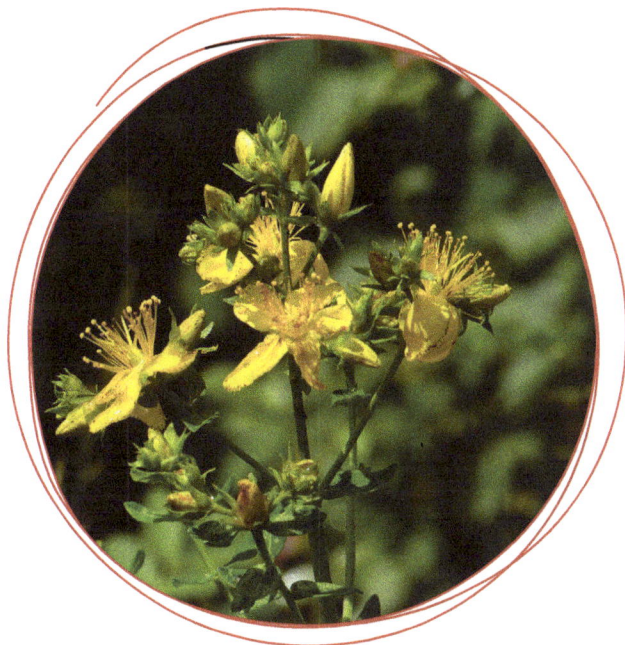

SOURCE: Wikimedia. Common St. John's wort (Hypericum perforatum).
Photo by Ryan Hodnett.

Gotu Kola (Centella asiatica). Gota Kola is high in B vitamins, vitamin C, and antioxidants with wound healing, sedative, anxiolytic, and antidepressant properties. It has been shown to increase circulation and cognitive functioning and has been used as a remedy for fatigue, insomnia, anxiety, and depression. Gotu Kola is widely used in India to improve memory and extend longevity. Evidence indicates that it may help with social anxiety and obsessive-compulsive disorder (OCD) and to attenuate age-related decline in cognitive function and mood disorder in the healthy elderly. [18]

CAUTION: *Because of Gotu Kola's sedative qualities, it is not recommended using it in combination with anxiety or sleep medications.*

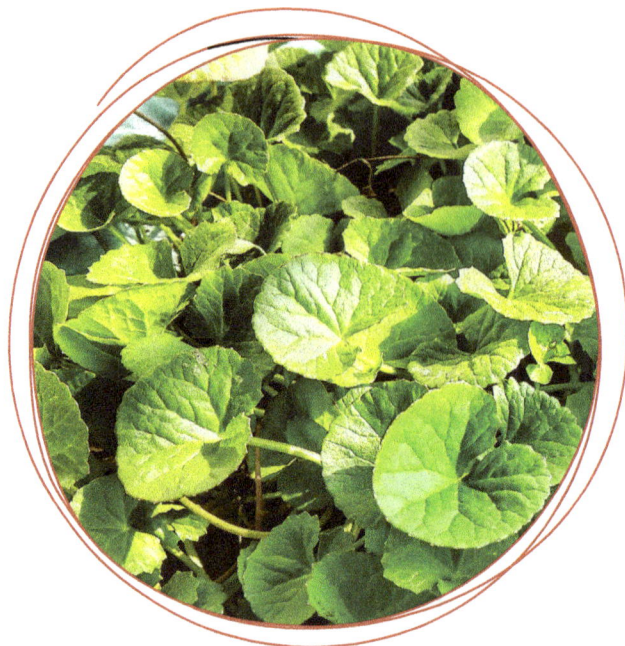

SOURCE: Wikimedia. Gotu Kola (Centella asiatica).
Photo by Shahidul Hasan Roman.

Kava Kava (Piper methysticum). Kava root has been used throughout the Pacific Ocean cultures of Polynesia for over 3,000 years, where it is an essential and integral part of life there. The roots of the kava plant are used to produce a drink with sedative and anesthetic properties for relaxation without disrupting mental clarity. Historically known as a peaceful euphoriant, kava creates a general feeling of well-being, induces a feeling of peace, relaxation, and contentment, enhances mental alertness, concentration and memory, reduces inhibitions, and makes people more sociable. It has been used in folk medicine as a natural antidepressant. Unlike alcohol, kava does not stimulate aggression or lead to hangover. Kava can be used on an as-needed basis for anxiety, panic attacks, or racing mind with no fear of addiction or change to one's personality. [19]

Much disinformation has been spread concerning kava and liver toxicity. According to researcher Jerome Sarris, of Australia's University of Queensland, kava has been used in the Pacific Islands where it has grown for centuries without evidence of liver problems. The reports of liver damage have widely been dismissed. Historically, the root only has been used safely for consumption. There has not been a single reported incident of kava liver damage from any products made solely from the plant's roots.

CAUTION: *Avoid the leaves, stems, and bark peelings from the aerial parts of the kava plant which contain toxic alkaloids and are never used in traditional kava preparations. Consult with a healthcare professional before using kava if you have had liver problems, frequently use alcoholic beverages, or are taking any medication. Kava Kava should not be taken with alcohol, barbiturates, anti-anxiety, anticoagulant, or antipsychotic medications.*

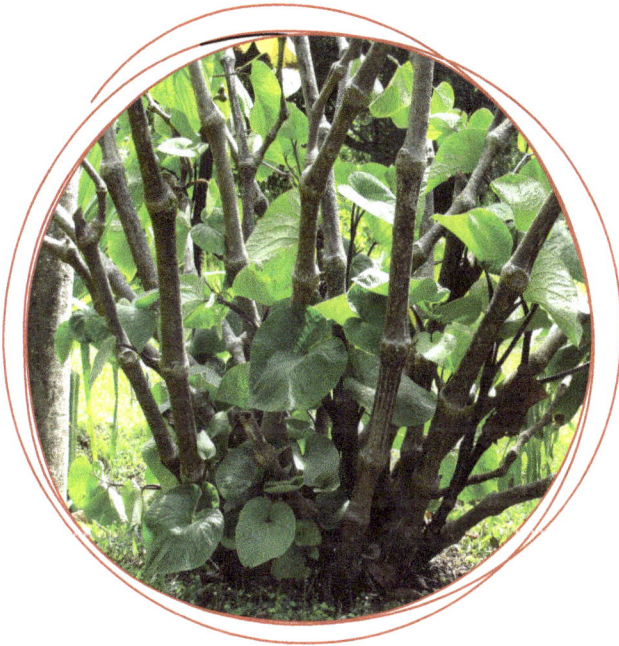

SOURCE: Piper methysticum-leaves stems and nodes.
Photo by Forest & Kim Starr.

Passionflower (Passiflora incarnata) has a tranquilizing effect on the nervous system and is indicated specifically for anxiety and insomnia. It works best for people with anxiety who also experience a lot of circular thinking or obsessive thoughts. With a reputation as a non-habit-forming medication for anxiety, passionflower has been indicated in preparations for alcohol, nicotine, and opiate withdrawal. It is high in flavonoids, niacin (B3), and glutamine and also contains calcium, iron, phosphorus, and quercetin.

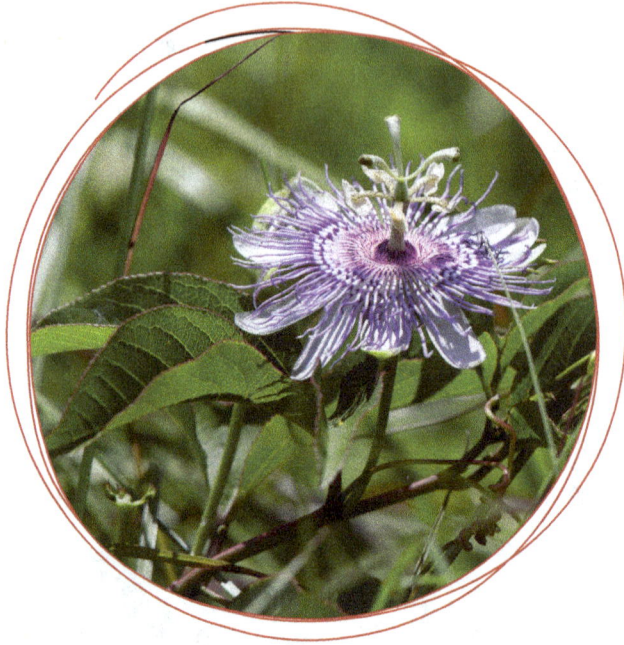

SOURCE: Wikimedia. Passionflower vine with purple bloom.
Photo by NASA/Bill White.

Lobelia (Lobelia inflata) is an anti-spasmodic stimulant and powerful nervine. It assists in removing obstruction and congestion in the body. Known as the "thinking herb," lobelia goes to whatever part of the body is ailing and treats it. Lobelia contains ascorbic acid, beta-carotene, calcium, magnesium, B vitamins, phosphorus, potassium, iron, selenium, and zinc.

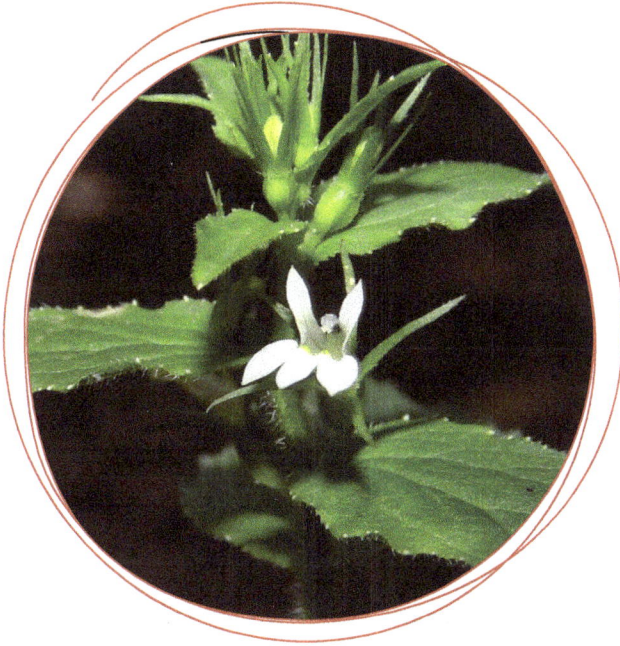

SOURCE: Wikimedia. Lobelia inflata flower.
Photo by Gordon C. Snelling.

Adaptogenic Herbs

Adaptogens are a class of herbs known to influence the body's response to physical, biological, chemical, and psychological stressors. Known for their calming energy, adaptogens have been shown to restore homeostasis, prevent adrenal burnout, increase vitality and energy, combat the effects of aging, regulate blood sugar, enhance the effectiveness of the liver, increase cellular energy, help the body to utilize oxygen more efficiently, and provide an increased sense of psychological and physical well-being. [20]

Only 50 years ago, the term "stress" was not part of the everyday vocabulary as it is today. Now in the twenty-first century, it has become an epidemic. We are moving faster, processing more information, and increasing the demand on our minds and bodies from excessive vibrational energy, radiation, and environmental toxins. Researchers estimate that between 60 to 90% of all illnesses are stress-related. When stress becomes chronic, there is a continual release of cortisol, resulting in inflammation, lowered immunity, impaired mental clarity, and the "fight, flight, or freeze" syndrome. By correcting imbalances in the neuroendocrine and immune systems, adaptogenic herbs normalize physiology that has been disturbed by prolonged stress.

Dr. Israel I. Brekhman, a Doctor of Medical Sciences, focused his career on unlocking the genetic secrets of plants and herbs to improve health and well-being. During his remarkable 45 years of research at the Naval Medical Academy of the U.S.S.R., Dr. Brekhman became the world authority on adaptogens and pioneered a vast scientific effort funded by the Russian government involving 1200 scientists and more than half a billion U.S. dollars to explore plant biological codes and their molecular structures. Since beginning his research in 1959, thousands of tests have been done on eleuthero and other herbal adaptogens. Hundreds of thousands of people have taken these herbs, which have shown remarkable effectiveness in preventing a variety of ailments and increasing stamina. [21]

After extensive research and testing, I have created a list of my favorite adaptogenic herbs that I have used personally and have recommended to countless others with great results. Before experimenting with any herbal remedies, consult with a qualified herbalist first. As always, if you are under medical care or taking any pharmaceutical medications, consult with your doctor before including herbal supplements into your diet.

Eleuthero (Eleutherococcus senticosus), formerly known as Siberian ginseng, eleuthero is indigenous to Siberia and northeastern China, where it has been used for over 2,000 years as a longevity tonic to increase vitality and resistance to stress. Eleuthero is the most intensely studied adaptogen, with over 40 years of clinical and practical research. And the results are astounding. Eleuthero promotes psychological and physical well-being, prevents adrenal burnout, boosts concentration, memory, and focus. It enhances the effectiveness of the liver, blood-sugar regulation, and DNA repair. It protects the body against environmental toxins, chemotherapy, and radiation. [22]

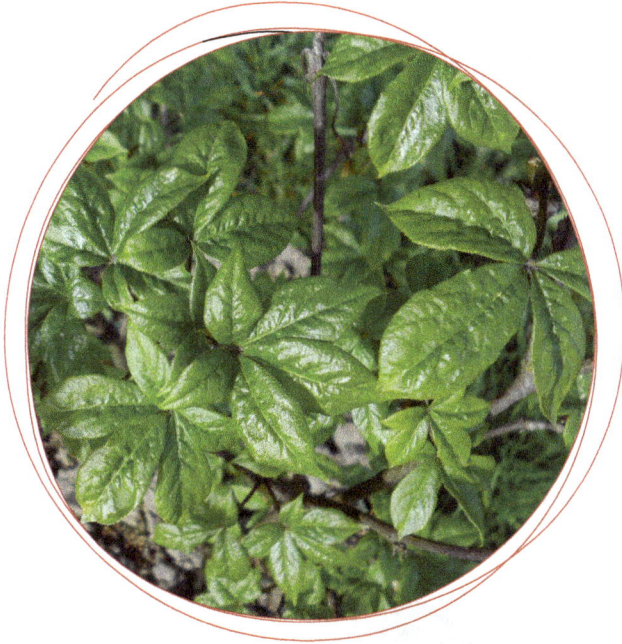

SOURCE: Wikimedia. Eleuthero (Eleuterococcus senticosus).
Photo by Salicyna.

Rhodiola (Rhodiola rosea) has been used for hundreds of years in Asia and Eastern Europe to enhance physical and mental performance. In Russia and Scandinavia, Rhodiola is commonly prescribed for treating fatigue, improving work performance, alleviating depression, and improving resistance to both physical and psychological stress. Rhodiola has been used by millions of Russians, including the Russian Olympic team, cosmonauts, and as a treatment for radiation exposure after the Chernobyl accident.

The Journal of The American Botanical Council, HerbalGram, published an Overview on Rhodiola rosea in 2002 based on more than one hundred Russian studies on the plant and its effects on health. The overview reported proven benefits of Rhodiola's use for the nervous, endocrine, cardiovascular, and reproductive systems and for its anti-cancer effects. The overview also described cases of improved mental and emotional health due to Rhodiola's use in patients who had not benefited from other interventions, including drugs and psychotherapy. [23]

Rhodiola lowers cortisol levels, promotes energy and stamina, and improves athletic performance and endurance. It is calming to the emotional system while energizing the brain's cognitive functions. Rhodiola has demonstrated a remarkable ability to enhance cellular energy metabolism, which decreases with age and causes most degenerative diseases. Rhodiola stimulates the release of dopamine, norepinephrine, and serotonin into ascending pathways in the brain that activate the cerebral cortex, stimulating analyzing, evaluating, calculating, and planning functions. The stimulant effect then moves to the prefrontal cortex, where it contributes to memory functions, including encoding, sorting, storage, and retrieval. Rhodiola has an impressive track record for reducing stress-induced fatigue and mild to moderate depression and significantly improving generalized anxiety disorder (GAD) symptoms. [24, 25]

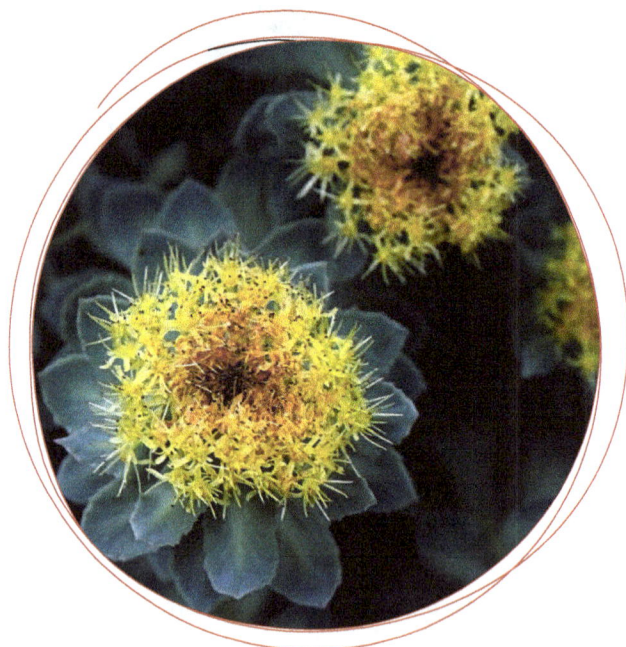

SOURCE: Wikimedia. Rosenwurz (Rhodiola rosea) 5727.
Photo by Hedwig Storch.

Ashwagandha (Withania somnifera) is the most frequently prescribed tonic herb in Ayurvedic medicine. Often referred to as "Indian ginseng,"

Ashwagandha has been studied with great interest by medical researchers and is reputed to increase energy and endurance, promote longevity, calm the mind, enhance mental function, support sexual vitality, strengthen immune function, reduce brain-cell degeneration, regulate blood sugar, and encourage restful sleep. Additionally, it helps the body overcome imbalances caused by mental or physical stress, poor diet, environmental toxins, or lack of sleep.

Scientific studies support ashwagandha's ability to protect brain cells against the effects of anxiety and depression. Oral administration of ashwagandha showed anxiety-relieving effects similar to those achieved by anti-anxiety and antidepressant prescription medications. Ashwagandha has powerful antioxidant properties that seek and destroy the free radicals associated with aging and disease. The Institute of Natural Medicine at the Toyama Medical and Pharmaceutical University in Japan has conducted extensive research into the brain benefits of ashwagandha and concluded that ashwagandha extract helps to reconstruct networks of the nervous system, making it a potential treatment for neurodegenerative diseases such as Alzheimer's. [26, 27]

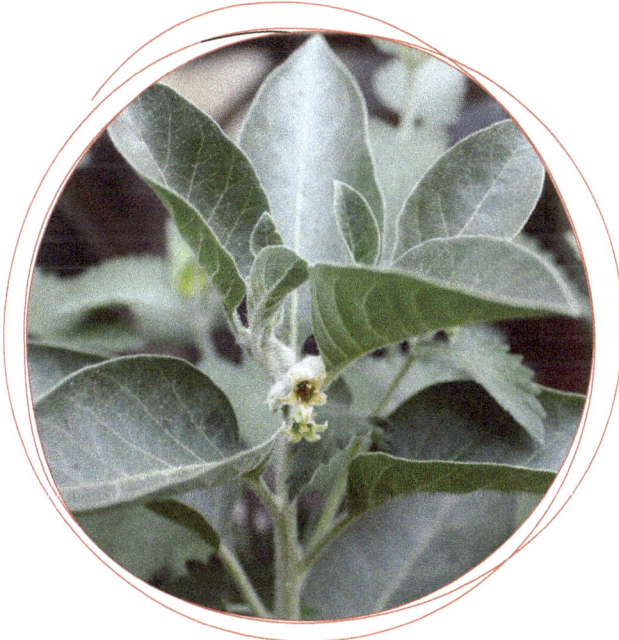

SOURCE: Wikimedia. Flowering ashwagandha plant
Photo by Wowbobwow12

Maca (Lepidium meyenii) grows in central Peru in the high plateaus of the Andes mountains and has been cultivated as a vegetable crop in Peru for at least 3000 years. It was highly prized by Incan warriors to increase stamina, boost libido, and combat fatigue. Maca contains 55 phytochemicals that are known to have vitality-enhancing effects in the body. The plant provides vitamins A, B, C, and D and is rich in minerals, with high concentrations of calcium, magnesium, iron, silica, manganese, copper, and zinc. Maca has been used to increase stamina, athletic performance, and memory. [28]

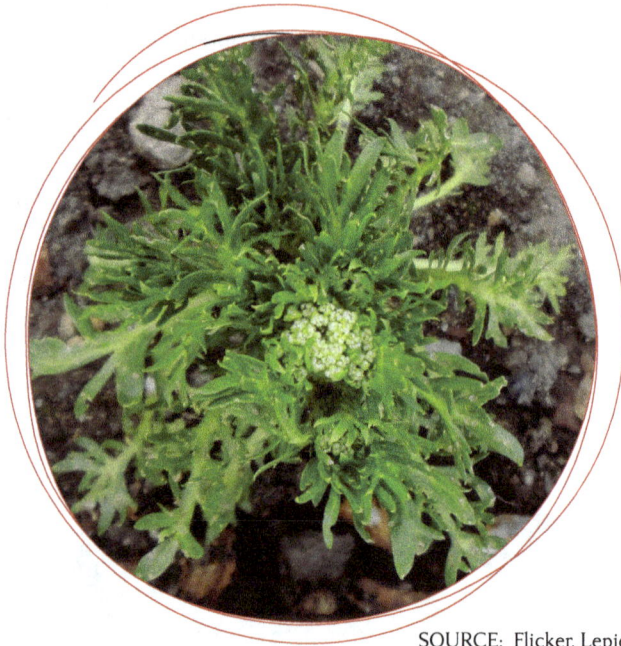

SOURCE: Flicker. Lepidium meyenii
Photo by Vahe Martirosyan

Schisandra Berries (Schisandra chinensis) was first recorded in the "Shennong Herbal Classic" more than 2000 years ago as a hepatoprotective drug in traditional Chinese medicine and has been an official drug in the Russian Pharmacopeia since 1961. It has been used safely for thousands of years as an anti-aging tonic, believed to increase stamina and mental clarity and fight fatigue and stress.

Laboratory experiments coupled with clinical trials in China confirm that schisandra helps improve brain efficiency, increase work capacity, mildly stimulate the central nervous system, improve reflexes, build strength, and increase endurance in healthy individuals. It is also said to help energize RNA and DNA molecules to rebuild cells. Research attributes the herb's medicinal effects to more than 40 compounds known as lignans called schisandrins. Studies have demonstrated schisandra's ability to make the enzyme, glutathione peroxidase, which deactivates several types of toxic free radicals that attack the outer membranes of the liver cells. Additionally, schisandra has been used for protecting against radiation, boosting energy at the cellular level, counteracting the effects of sugar, and improving the health of the adrenal glands. [29], [30]

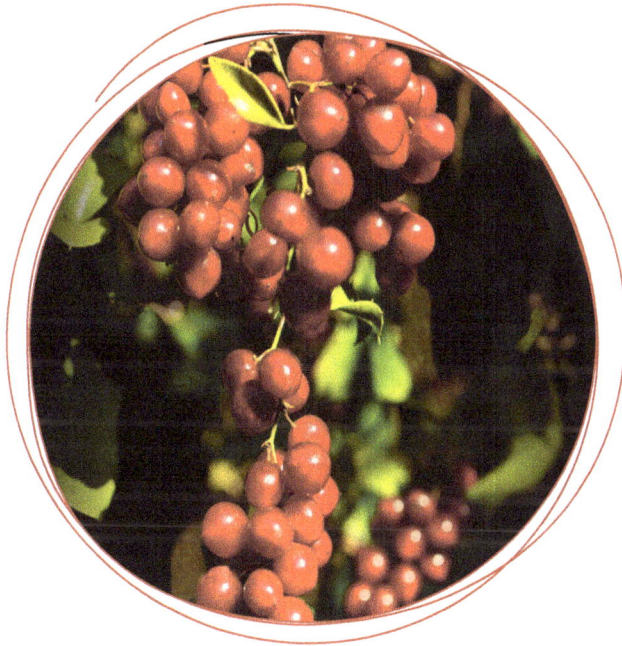

SOURCE: pxhere.com. Schisandra Berries
Photo by Marina del Castell

An herbalist can help you to determine which herbs and dosages may be best for you and to ensure that you are getting the purest form of herbs. It is not recommended that you combine herbs that have a calming effect with antidepressant medications. Consult with your doctor if you are taking prescription medications

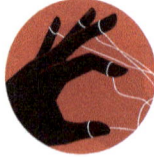

Chapter Five

HABITS THAT FEED YOUR SOUL

There is an intricate connection between the physical and emotional components of health and wellness. Trauma to your physical body can manifest emotionally, and emotional trauma (known or unknown) can be expressed in your physical body. This chapter will review some physical modalities that can help to release blockages, increasing energy flow, and enhancing well-being.

Exercise

Motion affects emotion. Exercise has been shown to have an antidepressant and anti-anxiety effect on mood. Studies show intervals of intense physical activity increase serotonin, feel-good endorphins, and other neurochemicals that decrease anxiety and increase pleasure.

Bursts of high-intensity anaerobic activity are one of the most efficient ways to achieve the greatest cardiovascular benefit to your heart while burning fat and losing weight. Known as HIIT (high-intensity interval training), Peak 8 Fitness, or Burst Fitness, this simple system involves exercising to your maximum capacity (15 to 20 seconds) and then allowing your body to recover fully to perform at 100% again. This cycle is then repeated to complete eight sets. [1] High-intensity interval training can delay aging by increasing the production of human growth hormone (HGH), which promotes muscle growth, reduces body fat, creates firmer skin, and creates more energy for improved athletic performance.

Weightlifting and resistance training can also boost mood without increasing heart rate. A study published in JAMA Psychiatry showed that resistance training significantly reduces symptoms of depression for those with mild to moderate depression. [2]

Exercising with others offers the additional emotional benefit of social- izing. Activities like hiking, dancing, biking, and group exercises release feel-good endorphins, especially when enjoyed with others.

Anything that gets you moving can be beneficial for your mood. Take things slowly if you are just starting out, and increase activity gradually to avoid injury.

Grounding

When the body is grounded, through physical contact with the earth, its electrical potential becomes equalized with the electrical potential of the Earth, releasing trapped electromagnetic energy in the body. When this stagnant charge is trapped in the body, it can lead to inflammation and increased cortisol secretion. Cortisol is the stress hormone that is released into the body when you become worried, fearful, or anxious and triggers the "fight, flight, or freeze" mechanism of the sympathetic nervous system. When cortisol remains high, it can contribute to sleep disorders, hypertension, cardiovascular disease, autoimmune diseases, blood sugar irregularity, and mood disorders.

Also known as earthing, grounding is a simple and effective way to normalize cortisol secretion and reduce inflammation and the chance of developing a chronic disease. Other benefits of grounding include better sleep, reduced pain, less stress, normalization of circadian rhythms and the function of the autonomic nervous system, decreased blood viscosity (associated with stroke and cardiovascular issues), faster recovery from injury or disease, reduction of primary indicators of osteoporosis, improvement of glucose regulation, and more efficient immune responses to trauma. [3, 4]

Chiropractic

Chiropractic doctors focus on preventing, diagnosing, and conservatively caring for spine-related disorders and joint issues. Chiropractic alignment restores joint function and supports the nervous system. New studies confirm the effectiveness of chiropractic care in relieving certain mental health symptoms while relieving tension, creating relaxation, and improving sleep. Studies show that following a chiropractic adjustment, your body triggers hormones that positively impact nervous system functioning. These include neurotensin, which neutralizes stress-induced pain; oxytocin, which enhances neuro-communication and promotes feelings of social bonding; and cortisol, which helps block pain resulting from inflammation. [5]

Massage

Massage is therapy for the body and the mind. Physically, it reduces muscle tension and pain and increases lymphatic flow. The mental health benefits include reduced anxiety, stress, and depression, improved mood, and increased energy levels. [6]

Tapping

Tapping, also known as Emotional Freedom Technique (EFT), is a powerful healing technique proven to effectively resolve a range of issues, including stress, anxiety, phobias, emotional disorders, chronic pain, weight control, and limiting beliefs. EFT does this by accessing the amygdala, the part of your brain that initiates your body's "fight, flight, or freeze" reaction to fear. Tapping is based on the combination of Ancient Chinese acupressure and modern psychology. The practice consists of tapping with your fingertips on specific meridian points while focusing on negative emotions or physical sensations. Doing this helps calm the nervous system, rewire the brain to respond in healthier ways, and restore the body's balance of energy. [7]

Laughter

On average, children laugh 10,000 times a week, while adults laugh an average of 5 times a week. How and when did we lose our sense of humor?

Anatomy of an Illness was the first book written by a patient that addressed the benefit of taking charge of your own health. When Norman Cousins was diagnosed with a crippling and irreversible disease and told that he had one chance in 500 of recovery, he collaborated with his physician to use his powers of laughter, courage, and tenacity to reverse his illness. His recovery program included massive intravenous doses of Vitamin C and self-induced bouts of laughter brought on by various television shows and comic films. In mobilizing his body's natural resources, Cousins proved what an effective healing tool the mind could be. [8]

Laughter has the unique ability to take you by surprise, producing an endorphin release that can lower your defenses, soften your perspectives, and make you more receptive to new ideas. Laughter is good medicine. Those with greater tendencies to cope using humor, report greater daily positive mood. These findings indicate that those who regain and maintain positive emotional states when faced with a stressful life experience can improve their immune function. [9]

> *A merry heart does good, like medicine, but a broken*
> *spirit dries the bones.*
>
> Proverbs 17:22

Creative Expression

Music, art, drama, dance, painting, sculpture, design, poetry, writing, gardening, sewing, and many other forms of artistic expression can lift and energize your mood. Activities that require thought and creativity stimulate brain activity and release joy within you and to those around you. What creates joy for you? Make room for that in your life to feed your soul.

Sound

Sound frequencies can elevate your emotions or bring them down. This principle applies to anything broadcasted in the air, over the airwaves, or through electronic devices as a sound, spoken message, or musical form. Sound frequencies can create a range of emotions such as fear, agitation, joy, melancholy, and anger—often without your awareness of the source. The Bible gives a great example of this. When an evil spirit tormented King Saul, he would summon David to play the harp. Saul would become refreshed and well when David played, and the distressing spirit would depart from him (I Samuel 16:23).

Prayer and Meditation

Connecting with your Creator through conversation, meditation, and listening for his voice can provide peace, wisdom, revelation, and guidance for all areas of your life. Being mindful, grateful, and declaring God's truths can transform and heal your body and soul. Journaling these experiences can serve as helpful reminders when you need encouragement later on.

Community and Giving

There is no lasting joy in living for yourself. When you have the nature of God within you, it is natural to want to give to others. When you are lacking or have a need, consider giving to someone else what you need. Giving time, money, energy, or emotional support shifts the focus from yourself and onto others. Giving generates a spirit of gratitude and activates the spiritual law of sowing and reaping (Galatians 6:7).

IT IS WELL WITH MY SOUL
A Story of Resilience and State of Mind

At the very height of his financial and professional success, Horatio Spafford, a wealthy Chicago lawyer, and his wife Anna suffered the tragic loss of their young son. Shortly thereafter, in 1871, the Great Chicago Fire destroyed almost every real estate investment Spafford had.

In 1873, Spafford scheduled a boat trip to Europe in order to give his wife and daughters a much-needed vacation and time to recover from the tragedy. He sent his wife and daughters ahead of him while he remained in Chicago to take care of some unexpected last-minute business. Several days later, he received notice that his family's ship had encountered a collision, and all four of his daughters drowned; only his wife had survived.

With a heavy heart, Spafford boarded a boat to meet with his grieving wife in England. When he reached the location where their boat went down, Horatio penned the words to what would become one of the most famous songs of faith. For more than a century, the tragic story of this one man has given hope to countless thousands that found comfort in those words, later set to music, "It Is Well With My Soul."

A situation like this could easily destroy a man. However, Spafford chose to declare, "it is well with my soul." He rose above the visible circumstances and set his eyes on the unseen. [10]

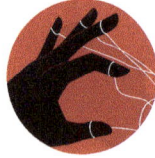

Chapter Six

THE WAR
FOR YOUR SOUL

Human beings have a great capacity for sticking to
false beliefs with great passion and tenacity.

— Bruce Lipton, *The Biology of Belief*

Your individual beliefs, based on your interpretation of life events, create your current reality. Your foundational beliefs are formed during your earliest observations of those closest to you. Because these beliefs are assimilated subconsciously, they are incorporated into your belief system without questioning their validity. How your brain processes information from life events is as unique to you as your fingerprints or the patterns in the iris of your eyes. Even those who share a life experience often interpret the situation differently, resulting in unique conclusions.

Your core beliefs are formed subconsciously during important events in your life. These events tend to have strong emotions (positive or negative) attached to them, which imprints the experience, feelings, and subsequent beliefs in your mind. Future events are then filtered through this established belief system, which influences your decisions and creates your current reality. This connection happens quickly and automatically, usually without your awareness. When these associations are reinforced over time, they become your foundational beliefs.

False beliefs are often at the root of emotional suffering. Left unchallenged, these lies can accumulate and create instability in your soul that can steal your peace, interfere with your relationships, and keep you from fulfilling your divine purpose. Once you understand the driving force behind negative emotions and reactions, you can challenge those beliefs and receive revelation that sets you free.

It takes great humility and a committed desire to grow in truth. This journey cannot be motivated by wanting others to be changed. By accepting personal responsibility, you can uncover your core beliefs, examine their validity, and receive transformational truth, even if those around you never change. There is an emotional battle for your soul. A sound mind is the goal, and your beliefs hold the key.

Science and Belief Systems

Only a generation ago, the scientific community assured us that brain cells, unlike other cells of the body, could not regenerate and would only decline in quality and quantity with age. In the mid-1990s, Dr. Bruce Lipton challenged this theory with his research into epigenetics, a rapidly growing area of science that focuses on the processes determining when individual genes are turned on or off. Today, it is widely accepted that the brain is alive and can be repaired and even improved as we age. In his groundbreaking book, *The Biology of Belief,* Dr. Lipton shows scientifically that life is not controlled by DNA alone, as originally believed. It is a symbiotic collaboration of nature (genes) and nurture (epigenetics). Research in epigenetics has shown that DNA blueprints passed down through genes are not permanently set at birth. Environmental influences, including nutrition, stress, and emotions can modify these genes, and modifications can be passed on to future generations.[1]

DNA is the blueprint, but it is your interpretation of the signals received from your environment and the resulting beliefs that determine the expression of your DNA. I love when science catches up the everlasting truth of God's Word!

> As a man thinks in his heart, so is he.
>
> Proverbs 23:7

Dr. Lipton summarizes these findings when he states, "I was exhilarated by the new realization that I could change the character of my life by changing my beliefs. I was instantly energized because I realized that there was a science-based path that would take me from my job as a perennial 'victim' to my new job as 'co-creator' of my destiny."[2] Can I get an "Amen?"

Conscious vs. Subconscious Beliefs

Human beings have the incredible capability to hold two opposing beliefs simultaneously—one on the conscious level and the other on the subconscious level. It is possible to believe something logically while feeling something contrary at your core. Both levels of belief serve an important purpose and can be used for your benefit. The conscious mind represents those elements that contribute to your personal identity, such as creativity, problem-solving, planning, and rationalization and is in control about 5% of the time. The subconscious mind is a million times more powerful and controls 95% of your life experiences.

You are continually evaluating life's events through your established belief system. When you encounter new experiences, your subconscious mind draws upon your reservoir of past experiences to interpret the situation. When your mind determines a current event to be similar to an earlier event, it will default to the subsequent feelings and beliefs attached to the historical event. If your interpretation is wrong, you can live your life based upon a lie that not only feels true, but the outcome will likely be the same as if it were true. Life will confirm what you believe to be true—the inevitable "self-fulfilling prophesy."

This association process is by divine design to help you navigate life's unknowns by drawing upon the knowledge and experiences that you have accumulated over time so that you can quickly assess a situation, calculate risks, and make quick decisions when necessary. This is especially useful in situations perceived to be physically or emotionally dangerous. In the process of rapidly assimilating volumes of valuable information, you are also embracing the impressions and beliefs of those around you. Once you accept the perceptions of others as truths, their perceptions become hardwired into your own brain and become your truths. By the age of six, your subconscious mind has determined your foundational beliefs, which are predominantly limiting and disempowering.[3]

These two belief systems are often at odds with one another and can cause confusion and distress. During times of emotional upheaval, your default reaction will be based on your subconscious, experiential beliefs. When core beliefs oppose logical beliefs, it creates an imbalanced emotional state. For example, I can logically believe that God will never leave me or forsake me while simultaneously feeling alone and abandoned. The Bible describes this as a "double-minded" man (James 1:4–8).

The capacity of the conscious mind to override the subconscious mind's preprogrammed behaviors is the foundation of free will. Through awareness and intentional mindfulness, the self-conscious mind can observe programmed behavior, evaluate it, and consciously decide how to respond. [4]

Disintegration to Transformation

From my earliest childhood memories, I felt deep sadness, loneliness, and abandonment. The ache in my heart was so familiar that I never questioned why I felt this way. It was just a part of me, my familiar dark companion. I was unaware of how much this affected me, not only as a child, but into my adult life.

Looking back now from a perspective of truth, I realize that my childhood and identity had been hijacked. My tiny world was turned on its axis as I embraced an adult-sized burden I would never be able to bear or resolve. I craved acceptance from everyone to feel validated, which resulted in becoming a people pleaser, often at my own expense. I was drawn to helping others in emotional pain, unaware of my own unresolved trauma.

My childhood wounds were expressed in adult ways that were great traits externally—dependable, responsible, and organized—but the subconscious motivation beneath them was to avoid unexpected catastrophes and remain in control. This resulted in increasing anxiety as I took on the responsibilities of the world.

I later learned that time did not heal the emotional wounds that I carried. Truth did. As I learned to identify the beliefs that were anchored to my pain and as I allowed the Spirit of Truth to respond to those beliefs, the pain was permanently resolved.

And you shall know the truth, and the truth shall make you free.

John 8:32

PATHWAYS TO TRUTH

Truth can come to us in various and unique ways. I recognize truth when it resonates deeply within my soul and is wise beyond my human capacity. Here are some ways that I have been changed by truth. Perhaps some resonate with you.

God's Word is the gold standard of truth—everlasting and unchanging. As you read and meditate on God's Word, the written Word (logos) becomes a living (rhema) Word that can transform your mind.

Logos represents words. A rhema word is a life-changing revelation that happens in a moment.

> *For the word of God is living and powerful, and sharper than any two-edged sword, piercing even to the division of soul and spirit, and of joints and marrow, and is a discerner of the thoughts and intents of the heart.*
>
> Hebrews 4:12

Divine revelation is a personal unveiling of information. It can come in the form of a word, message, image, or simply a "knowing" that you recognize as truth.

> *However, when He, the Spirit of truth, has come, He will guide you into all truth; for He will not speak on His own authority, but whatever He hears He will speak; and He will tell you things to come.*
>
> John 16:13

Prophetic words received directly from the Spirit of Truth or from another person. You may not know the impact or truth in the moment, but it is proven over time.

Wisdom from others, such as a parent, friend, mentor, counselor, teacher, or pastor. Discernment is essential in evaluating these messages. You do not have to receive everything that is spoken to you, over you, or about you.

Personal experience can be a painful but effective teacher. Some things are only learned through experience.

Messages all around us often come in unexpected ways through stories, movies, art, nature, and beauty.

Dreams come from various sources and for different reasons, and most often cannot be taken literally. Dreams help your mind sort through all the information taken in through your senses every day. Your dreams can also provide divine revelation and reveal spiritual messages. We can also be deceived by the messages we receive. It takes discernment and wisdom to filter truth from lies.

Here are some examples from the scriptures:

> And Pharaoh said to Joseph, "I have had a dream, and there is no one who can interpret it. But I have heard it said of you that you can understand a dream, to interpret it."
>
> Genesis 41:15

> Then He said, "Hear now My words: If there is a prophet among you, I the Lord make Myself known to him in a vision; I speak to him in a dream.
>
> Numbers 12:6

> At Gibeon the Lord appeared to Solomon in a dream by night; and God said, "Ask! What shall I give you?"
>
> I Kings 3:5

> Then the secret was revealed to Daniel in a night vision.
>
> Daniel 2:19

> For God may speak in one way, or in another, yet man does not perceive it. In a dream, in a vision of the night, when deep sleep falls upon men, while slumbering on their beds, then He opens the ears of men, and seals their instruction.
>
> Job 33:14–16

> Then, being divinely warned in a dream that they should not return to Herod, they departed for their own country another way.
>
> Matthew 2:12

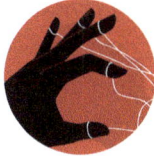

Chapter Seven

ENTANGLEMENTS

*We have made lies our refuge, and under falsehood
we have hidden ourselves.*

Isaiah 28:15b

Unresolved emotional pain can hinder you from fulfilling the destiny God has for your life. Emotional clutter subconsciously clamors for your attention, triggered by situations, people, or things your brain connects to unresolved wounds. Engaging in various forms of physical or mental distraction is often the behavior of choice for dealing with emotional turmoil. These comforting solutions can create entanglements that hinder you from resolving internal conflict and finding genuine peace. What appears to be the problem (addictions, habits, and sinful behaviors) may be your solution to managing pain and emotional stress.

One of my favorite visual analogies of the cycle of unresolved pain involves Otis, the endearing town drunk from the Andy of Mayberry television series. Numbing out through alcohol was Otis' solution of choice, and when the intoxication wore off, the inevitable burden of guilt and shame would set in. Otis would then turn himself in to the police department and put himself in jail, where he served the sentence he believed he deserved. The interesting thing is, the door was never locked; the keys just dangled on the outside of the cell door, and dear Otis could leave at any time. Only his guilt and self-condemnation kept him there. This cycle would repeat the next time Otis needed to silence his familiar pain.

If you recall from the previous chapter, 95% of your reactions are automatic and subconscious. These responses, reinforced over time and held in place by your beliefs, can serve as a quick fix to emotional pain. Through intentional awareness (the 5% realm), you can allow your pain to reveal what you believe and examine the validity of those beliefs. As you exercise this process, you will learn to recognize your protective mechanisms and allow the Spirit of Truth to untangle them before they can choke out the truth (Matthew 13:7).

Here are some common entanglements to consider.

Anger

Anger is a protective emotion, often the first emotion to show up and make the most noise to protect you from feeling the deeper, more vulnerable emotions under the surface. Anger can be toward a person, situation, God, or yourself. Anger may present initially because of truth but is held in place long-term by lies that result from holding on to it. Look behind the anger to identify the real emotion hiding there.

Unforgiveness (toward God, others, and self)

> *And whenever you stand praying, if you have anything against anyone, forgive him, that your Father in heaven may also forgive you your trespasses. But if you do not forgive, neither will your Father in heaven forgive your trespasses.*
>
> Mark 11:25–26

Unforgiveness is one of the major roadblocks to receiving emotional freedom. Without close examination, you are often unaware of harboring this burden. Carrying around unforgiveness is like trying to run a race with a ball and chain around your ankle (Hebrews 12:1).

Unforgiveness keeps toxic feelings alive and keeps you connected with the person or event that initiated the offense. How often have you been instructed to just "let it go" when someone has betrayed you? Moreover, how often have you genuinely tried to do just that, with little or no lasting effect? When you forgive the offender without considering the weight of the offense, the negative feelings will resurface when future situations trigger your lingering pain. Jesus illustrates true forgiveness in a story about a servant who owed a debt too great ever to repay (Matthew 18:23–35). When they presented the debtor to the king, the king examined what the debtor owed but did not examine the debtor himself. He then chose to cancel the debt, which released the debtor. To experience permanent forgiveness, consider the weight of the offense—what someone did to you, what someone denied you, and the cost to you. Can you release that? If not, consider the belief that is causing your hesitation.[1]

Left unchallenged, unforgiveness can lead to bitterness and resentment. Unforgiveness can create an expectation toward people and circumstances that can result in a self-fulfilling prophecy in opposition to your heart's true desires. You will know you have achieved complete forgiveness when genuine compassion and peace replace the negative emotions of unforgiveness.

One of the most critical and neglected elements of forgiveness is toward yourself. When you cannot forgive yourself, you are choosing to believe that the sacrifice of Jesus is not enough to atone for you and that you must pay an additional cost to receive his perfect gift. Accepting undeserved forgiveness requires humility.

Anger toward God is never rooted in truth, and God does not need forgiveness. Your acknowledgment, repentance, and release of anger toward him are for your benefit.

Forgiveness is a gift to the giver.

Vows, Decisions, and Agreements

Vows are often made during times of stress, frustration, anger, or trauma and can provide a false sense of power and protection to help you cope with an unbearable situation. Your agreement with the vow may limit you in unknown ways. Once the vow has been identified and the belief anchoring the vow is uncovered, the truth can be received which eliminates the need for the self-limiting vow.

Words from Others

Social media/TV/movies/news: Be aware of how these information portals are feeding or harming your soul. What is the message and how does it make you feel and react?

Friends, family, colleagues, educators, pastors, mentors, spouses, and significant others may offer well-intended words of encouragement or advice based on their mistaken beliefs and fears, shifting your focus in the wrong direction. Be discerning about what messages you accept into your soul.

Curses are words intentionally spoken over others to control them or cause them harm. If you belong to Jesus, you can renounce and break any curse, known or unknown (Isaiah 54:17).

What you say about yourself has the most significant impact on your life. When the words of others cause you pain, it is often because of lies you already believe about yourself. When your beliefs align with whom God says you are, you will be kinder to yourself, and contrary opinions will not have power over you.

Protecting Others

Protecting those you care about can deter your healing. Sometimes when you begin the process of inner healing, it can widen the gap in your deepest relationships. You may subconsciously sabotage your progress to avoid this increased hostility in the relationship. Here are two examples that impacted me.

A mentor shared a story of limiting her own success. When she began to succeed in her acting career, she felt alienated from her "starving artist" friends, who bonded over their struggle. As a result, she was unknowingly self-sabotaging her success. Through emotional coaching, she became aware of this behavior and consciously decided to embrace her success, which led to her helping others do the same.

A friend once shared that the more her husband walked through his healing journey, the more offensive he became to her. In her mind, his trans-formation magnified her as the problem, and as a result, her shame increased. Fortunately, her husband was a patient man, and she eventually walked through her own healing journey with his love and support.

Sin Consciousness

Sin consciousness can become a roadblock to physical and emotional healing. The weight of unworthiness can make you feel disqualified to receive the grace of God, even though he desires to heal you. Consider the story of the paralytic and how Jesus forgave his sins when he was brought to him for physical healing (Matthew 9:1–8). By forgiving the man his sin, Jesus removed the mental roadblock and set the man up for a miracle. He was then able to receive the gift of healing fully.

Avoidance

Procrastinating, exhaustion, overwhelm, and other forms of numbing out can be defense mechanisms to avoid facing your pain. In a familiar Bible story, God told the prophet Jonah to go to the town of Nineveh to warn the people that they were about to be judged unless they repented of their wickedness. Instead, Jonah boarded a boat heading in another direction. When a wild storm came upon the boat, everyone was frantically trying to remedy the situation—except for the person responsible for the storm.

> *But the Lord sent out a great wind on the sea, and there*
> *was a mighty tempest on the sea, so that the ship was*
> *about to be broken up. Then the mariners were afraid;*

and every man cried out to his god and threw the cargo
that was in the ship into the sea, to lighten the load. But
Jonah had gone down into the lowest parts of the ship,
had lain down, and was fast asleep. So, the captain came
to him, and said to him, "What do you mean, sleeper?
Arise, call on your God; perhaps your God will consider
us, so that we may not perish.

Jonah 1:4–6

As the story continues, the waves are calmed only after Jonah is thrown overboard where he is swallowed by a huge fish. He remained there for three days and was then delivered by the fish onto the shores of Nineveh where he conceded to God's will. When Jonah warned the people, they repented and turned from their sin, and the city was spared.

Medications

Some medications can inhibit a person's ability to focus and feel, which are necessary for bringing subconscious memories into the conscious realm where they can be resolved.

Dissociation

Dissociation is an innate survival technique that allows you to survive a traumatic situation by disconnecting mentally. The dissociation happens initially to survive a traumatic event, but the dissociation that was helpful during the trauma is now creating its own set of problems. In severe cases, you can dissociate into a state of mental fragmentation that is called dissociative identity disorder (DID), formerly known as multiple personality disorder (MPD). These fragmented states are sometimes referred to as "alters," which are alternate personalities that are representations of the person's inner mental world. During traumatic life events, you are more vulnerable to believing lies that are then assimilated into your belief system. The mind may be able to keep these memories from your conscious awareness for a while but eventually, the effects of the event start permeating into your life in ways that are harder to ignore. Emotions are the bridge between the fragmented memory and your conscious awareness, and God's truth can restore what was lost during the traumatic incident.[2]

Soul Ties

A soul tie is a connection made between two people on a physical, emotional, or spiritual level that binds them together. These connections can be by choice or by force, are often made without your awareness, and can have a lasting effect, either positive or negative.

Some Examples of Soul Ties

The intimate connection between a husband and a wife creates a soul tie that God intended for us to have, where the two become one.

> *For this reason a man shall leave his father and mother*
> *and be joined to his wife, and the two shall become*
> *one flesh.*
>
> Matthew 19:5

Soul ties from prior intimate relationships can form an unstable foundation for future healthy relationships. I have witnessed amazing transformations in relationships when praying with those who have acknowledged and released these bonds.

Healthy relationships with friends and family can form healthy soul ties.

> *The soul of Jonathan was knit to the soul of David, and*
> *Jonathan loved him as his own soul.*
>
> I Samuel 18:1

When a child assumes the role of the parent in a family, it can result in an unstable bond between them. The parent is usually unaware of the role reversal. They may be unwilling or unable to fulfill their parenting role because of trauma, mental or physical illness, addiction, abandonment, divorce, or death.

Occult Involvement

Involvement in the occult can create dark entanglements in the soul, which can cause confusion and hinder emotional healing. People often encounter the occult in ways that may seem innocent and harmless. However, a lack of understanding in these areas does not prevent negative spiritual results. You can receive freedom and healing through self-examination, repentance, and releasing these holds.

What is your behavior of choice for dealing with emotional turmoil, and what belief holds it in place? When the lie maintaining your preferred solution is identified and replaced with the truth, that solution will no longer have power or be needed.

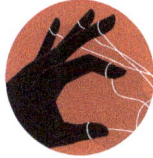

Chapter Eight

MIND RENEWAL

*He reveals deep and secret things; He knows what is
in the darkness and light dwells with Him.*

Daniel 2:22

How can you identify your deeply ingrained false beliefs and how can they be changed? Countless hours—that can quickly become years—have been spent with sincere intention, trying to convert wrong thinking into lasting truth, only to discover a life-long struggle between what you believe intellectually and what you feel emotionally in your heart. What you believe emotionally (true or not), especially during a crisis, will most likely determine your response to a situation. However, you can know the truth, and the truth will make you free (John 8:32).

Identifying the Lie

CAUTION: *The information presented does not apply to physical impairments in the body or brain that can create a disruption or distortion of cognitive functioning. Consulting with a medical doctor is imperative in those situations. Our focus will be on the emotional and spiritual roots of beliefs.*

You have an enemy whose mission is to kill, steal, and destroy, and his primary weapon is deception. Infamously known as "the father of lies" (John 8:44), this enemy torments you when your beliefs are aligned with his. Jesus is the Truth (John 14:6) and when he speaks into the place of emotional pain, the lie is replaced with the truth and the result is peace.

Most lies you believe fall into one of two categories: self-identity beliefs or state of being beliefs. What you feel reveals your heart belief. [1] Wrong beliefs may be expressed as anxiety, emotional unrest, lack of peace, an overreaction to situations or people, a distracted mind, circulating thoughts, feeling stuck, and being critical and judgmental of yourself or others.

Prayer, meditation, and learning to hear the voice of God are worthy investments in your emotional health. When you deliberately slow down and examine your thoughts and feelings, you can discover the beliefs that are anchoring your pain. As you receive truth in these areas, your mind is transformed.

Though time may lessen the emotional pain of past hurts and trauma, it may not heal the wound created during the event. A living rhema word from the Spirit of Truth has the power to displace the lie with truth and bring permanent healing. Though the memory remains the same, you now see it through the eyes of truth. Once truth has flooded that space, darkness can no longer reside there. The result of this supernatural encounter is genuine peace. As lies are removed, your carnal mind is transformed to the mind of Christ (Romans 8:6, Philippians 4:6–7). Spiritual revelation can save years of emotional struggle.

When beginning this process of mind renewal, a trained facilitator who has experience in this area can be a valuable mentor to you. You are often unaware of the ways that your mind subconsciously disrupts progress along the healing path, depending on the belief and strongholds surrounding that belief. As you work with a mentor and become familiar with the process of mind renewal, you will become equipped to identify emotional triggers in the moment and consciously deal with any wrong thinking before it becomes part of your core belief system.

Painful Emotions Rooted in Truth

Not all painful emotions are rooted in lies. Emotions such as disappointment, grief, sadness, regret, and anger can be based in truth when they are experienced for a season. You were created in the image of God and experience emotions just as he does. Unlike humans, God's emotions are always founded in truth. Here are some examples.

Jesus felt anguish in his soul, aware of the path ahead of him (John 12:27). However, he understood the truth and endured the cross for the joy set before him.

Jesus felt true abandonment. Most of his disciples left him when he was arrested and crucified (Matthew 26:4). He also suffered abandonment from his Father when he hung on the cross, receiving the full punishment for the sins of humankind.

> *And about the ninth hour Jesus cried out with a loud voice, saying, "Eli, Eli, lama sabachthani?" that is, My God, My God, why have You forsaken Me?*
> Matthew 27:46

Jesus felt love and deep sadness for Jerusalem.

> *O Jerusalem, Jerusalem, the one who kills the prophets and stones those who are sent to her! How often I wanted to gather your children together, as a hen gathers her chicks under her wings, but you were not willing!*
> Matthew 23:37

Jesus expressed grief when his friend Lazarus died.

> *Jesus wept.*
> John 11:35

Jesus displayed righteous anger when confronting the money changers in the temple.

> *Then Jesus went into the temple of God and drove out*
> *all those who bought and sold in the temple and*
> *overturned the tables of the money changers and the*
> *seats of those who sold doves.*
>
> Matthew 21:12

When we experience painful emotions that are based in truth, we can cast those burdens on the Lord and he will sustain us (Psalms 55:22).

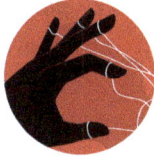

Chapter Nine

BEARING YOUR BROTHER'S BURDEN

God is not unjust; he will not forget your work
and the love you have shown him
as you have helped his people
and continue to help them.

Hebrews 6:10

Understanding how to support another person in their healing journey without rescuing them has been one of my most liberating areas of emotional wellness.

In the scriptures, the apostle Paul admonishes the Galatians to *"bear one another's burdens (barons) and so fulfill the law of Christ"* (Galatians 6:2). Later in verse five, he tells them that *"each one shall bear his own load (portion)."*

To clarify this seeming contradiction, we must understand the difference between a burden and a load.

A burden (Greek = *baros*) is something heavy pressing down on a person physically, emotionally, or spiritually—a crushing weight too big to be carried alone.

On the other hand, a load (Greek = *phortion*) refers to the troubles of this life, man's load of imperfections and sins; the portion that is the duty belonging to a specific person.

Therefore, Galatians 6:2 speaks of the relief someone needs while bearing a crushing weight, while verse five refers to the personal responsibility each of us has in the troubles of life.

By rescuing someone from their emotional pain, you may unknowingly keep them from receiving lasting freedom. They may feel relief initially, but if this cycle continues, they can become dependent on you as their source of relief. You may feel burdened and frustrated as they remain emotionally stuck in the same place.

Identifying what is your responsibility (sharing the burden) and what can be done by the person in pain (their load) is the first step to being a supportive friend. Are you more invested in this person's healing than they are? If so, this is a good time to step back and allow the other person to step up. Until they are willing to take ownership of their feelings and pain, you cannot help them. Focus on yourself and the work God wants to continue doing in you, and trust in God to do the work only he can do for others.

Second, consider any underlying reasons you may struggle to allow someone to stand on their own. What appears to be compassion can be a way to silence the negative voices in your own mind and avoid your own healing process.

Third, develop healthy boundaries. If the person in pain wants you to rescue them when they are in a crisis, continually blames others for their situation, and refuses to accept accountability, then stepping back may be a wise decision for you. Temporarily coming alongside someone to share their burden as they work through their healing is compassionate. Being their savior is not healthy for either of you. As always, if someone is in a crisis, refer them to a mental health professional.

Lastly, prioritize your own physical, emotional, and spiritual health. Those drawn to helping others are at a higher risk of becoming burned out over time. Unless you are intentional about your health and well-being, you can become overburdened helping others which can lead to anxiety, heart disease, diabetes, depression, and in extreme cases, suicide. The following statistics on rescue workers illuminate this point.

First responders, including police officers and firefighters, are more likely to die from suicide than in the line of duty, according to a recent study. In 2017, at least 103 firefighters and 140 police officers took their own lives, compared to the 93 firefighters and 129 police officers who died in the line of duty, the Ruderman Family Foundation reports. The mental health study cited PTSD and depression stemming from trauma exposure as factors contributing to higher-than-usual suicide rates.

Additionally, the recorded rates of suicide among first responders could be artificially low. The Firefighter Behavioral Health Alliance estimates that approximately 40% of firefighter suicides are reported. This could make the actual number of suicides in 2017 closer to 257—more than twice the number of firefighters who died in the line of duty. [1]

The following story provides a beautiful visual of helping a friend in a way they cannot help themselves.

> *They came to him, bringing a paralytic who was carried by four men. And when they could not come near him because of the crowd, they uncovered the roof where he was. When they had broken through, they let down the bed on which the paralytic was lying. When Jesus saw their faith, he said to the paralytic, "Son, your sins are forgiven you."*
>
> Mark 2:3–5

Jesus healed the man because of the faith of his friends. I love that. We can have faith for others when their burden is too great to have faith of their own. Friends were essential in getting the man to where he needed to be, but only Jesus could perform the miracle.

Nani's Miracle

More than 20 years ago, my mother-in-law was diagnosed with Stage 4 non-Hodgkin's lymphoma in multiple organs and was given three months at most to live. As the reality of this devastating news began to sink in, God's still, small voice reminded me of the faith my mother-in-law had shared with me many years earlier.

That same day, my family of five went to visit our dear Nani and together, we laid hands on her, anointed her with oil (Mark 6:13; James 5:14), renounced the cancer, and declared healing over her. As she looked up at me, I could see faith renewed in her eyes.

My daughter, who was in eighth grade at the time, put on a necklace from her Nani and told me she would not be removing it until Nani was healed. Several months later, Alexa came home from school and ecstatically told me, "Mom, I know Nani is healed because my necklace keeps falling off!"

Later that week, my mother-in-law called to tell us that the cancer was completely gone! I had her repeat it several times because I could hardly understand what she was saying with the shrill of excitement in her voice. It was true—there was no evidence of cancer anywhere. It would be 11 years, still cancer free, before our Nani would go to her eternal home.

I realize that stories like this can be very painful for those who did not receive the miracle in the way they had hoped and prayed.

In those situations, we grieve with those who are grieving and trust that God has a plan beyond our understanding. I hope this story encourages your faith and that we never stop praying for healing, deliverance, and restoration.

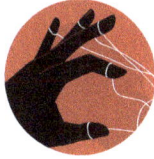

Chapter Ten

SPIRITUAL
TRANSFORMATION

*If I find in myself desires which nothing in this world can satisfy,
the only logical explanation is that I was
made for another world.*

— C. S. Lewis, *Mere Christianity*

Previous chapters addressed the assaults on the body and mind that can affect emotional stability. This chapter provides a glimpse into the vast realm of the spirit and how forces beyond the visible dimension or logical comprehension can improve or devastate mental health. The following insights are based on my personal revelation and beliefs.

God created you as a spirit being, possessing a soul, and living in a physical body. Each part influences the other. Your spirit is your intuition and conscience, the part of you that connects to your Creator, who is Spirit (John 4:24). The soul is your mind, will, emotions, senses, imagination, reasoning, and intellect. The body is your visible expression to the physical world and it is influenced by your spirit and soul (1 Thessalonians 5:23).

Your Creator longs to have a relationship with you and for you to be part of his plans in this temporary realm and for eternity. To restore the connection that was broken when sin entered the world, God sent his Son Jesus, fully God and fully man, as a perfect sacrifice to bridge the gap between you and a Holy, perfect God (John 3:16). This connection brings radical life and healing to your soul.

Conversely, dark spiritual forces are working to subvert that connection with spiritual counterfeits that can harm your soul.

> For we do not wrestle against flesh and blood, but
> against principalities, against powers, against the rulers
> of the darkness of this age, against spiritual hosts of
> wickedness in the heavenly places.
>
> Ephesians 6:12

Humility is the first step to everlasting life, acknowledging your need for a Savior. When you receive this gift of salvation through Jesus, your spirit is immediately regenerated, and a magnificent shift occurs in the spirit realm. Your mind begins transformation by God's Spirit, which can manifest in the restoration of your physical body (Romans 12:2; 2 Corinthians 3:18).

> Jesus said to him, "I am the way, the truth, and the life.
> No one comes to the Father except through Me."
>
> John 14:6

The reaction of the two criminals toward Jesus, as they hung on the cross alongside him, is a perfect portrayal of this choice. One man was offended by Jesus and blasphemed him with his dying breath, while the other man humbly acknowledged his sinful state and asked Jesus to "remember me when you come into your Kingdom." Jesus responded, "Assuredly, I say to you, today you will be with me in Paradise" (Luke 23:39–43). With those simple words, the man was fully forgiven and now lives eternally in heaven with Jesus.

*Therefore, if anyone is in Christ, he is a new creation;
old things have passed away; behold, all things have
become new.*

2 Corinthians 5:17

Above anything else you gain from this book, your relationship with your Creator and accepting the salvation he has freely provided for you through his Son, is the most important message within these pages. Let me know if you have made this decision while reading this book. I would love to talk with you more about your decision.

Dad

My dad is a beautiful example of God's unconditional love and grace. He created some of my fondest childhood memories, and I always felt loved by him. He supported my backyard theatrical performances, built the most amazing treehouse for me in the woods behind our house, planned every detail of my surprise birthday party, set up a "classroom" in the basement with subject workbooks so I could "teach" all my friends, and confronted a horrible teacher at school that made me cry. Unfortunately, those wonderful memories were overshadowed by sinister events embedded in my young mind when dad regularly came home intoxicated. I was terrified of the alcoholic persona, and I knew he wasn't my real dad.

My life was suspended for years as I remained in a state of alert. Dad continued to drink while neglecting to pay the bills, so we were evicted from our home when I was in fourth grade. My mom, sister, brother, and I moved into a small apartment on the South Side of Pittsburgh, where we were surrounded by a large, loving, and supportive family. As much as I did not want my dad around and feared he would harm my mother, my heart ached deeply when we left him behind. He continued to drink and spiral downhill. There was a painful hole in my heart, and I doubted I would ever see him again.

Ten years later, my sister, brother, and I reunited with our dad. By then he was sober and I started to see the real dad that I knew and always loved. Our reunion lasted five years. During the last three years of his life, dad battled throat cancer. It was heartbreaking, we were just getting to know each other again. God knew my dad's life was coming to an end and, in his magnificent graciousness, he made a way for us to be united again and for dad to be spiritually transformed before entering eternity.

At the end of dad's battle with cancer, he was anxious and frustrated as he lay in the hospital bed, unable to communicate because his voice box and part of his tongue had been removed. He desperately tried to write out his words, but they were illegible scribbles. I felt helpless and was unable to comfort him. Eventually, he slipped into a coma and remained in that state for hours.

While I was alone with him, he suddenly awoke from his coma—eyes wide, face illuminated and full of joy—lifting his body from the bed and pointing across the room, signaling to me, "look, look!" Dad was crossing over and could clearly see in the physical and spiritual realms simultaneously. Still full of joy, he drifted back into his coma and left this world shortly after. It has been decades since then, and I am still in awe when I remember that sacred moment. God allowed me to see my dad ecstatic and joyful as he crossed over into eternity. What an amazing parting gift.

Precious in the sight of the Lord is the death of His saints.

Psalm 116:15

SCIENCE AND SPIRITUAL BELIEFS

It is our interpretation of life events and
the resulting beliefs that determine
the expression of our DNA

— Bruce Lipton, *The Biology of Belief*

Why are your spiritual beliefs important and how do they affect your emotional health? Thousands of scientific articles are written every year about the impact of religion and spirituality on health and longevity. Here are some interesting conclusions from a few of them.

In his journey to understand the effects of belief on biology and behavior, Dr. Bruce Lipton, once a self-proclaimed, hyper-rational, religion-phobic scientist, concluded that "a person's belief in the afterlife has a substantial effect on their health and wellbeing." [1]

After reviewing more than 600 studies on the effects of religion and spirituality on mental health, Dr. Harold G. Koenig, Professor of Medicine at Duke University, concluded that people who are more religious/spiritual (R/S) have better mental health and adapt more quickly to health problems than those who are less spiritually inclined. Of the Big Five personality traits most commonly measured, R/S persons tend to score lower on neuroticism, especially low on psychoticism, higher on extraversion and openness to experience, and especially high on agreeableness and conscientiousness. Firmly held spiritual beliefs give meaning to difficult life circumstances and provide a sense of purpose resulting in less depression, lower stress, less anxiety, greater well-being, and more positive emotions. Positive emotions include happiness, hope, optimism, high self-esteem, and a sense of control over life resulting in traits such as altruism, compassion, gratitude, and forgiveness. One of the most impressive results of Koenig's research is regarding mortality. Of 121 studies examined, 68% found that greater R/S predicted significantly greater longevity. [2]

Data from the 2016 General Social Survey (GSS) of the Journal of Spirituality in Mental Health was analyzed to understand the relationship between Americans' religious and spiritual beliefs and behaviors and their mental health. Spiritual/religious beliefs and behaviors measured included afterlife beliefs, belief in God, prayer, service attendance, and self-perceived religiosity and spirituality. The most consistent predictor of enhanced mental health and well-being was more frequent service attendance. [3]

The Journal of Spirituality in Mental Health conducted a research study investigating the possible relationship between religious coping styles and spiritual well-being with two psychological variables: anxiety and depression. The study found that individuals reporting higher levels of religiosity and spiritual well-being may also experience a reduction in mental and emotional illness. [4]

Positive psychology is the latest classification of Western psychology, following the disease model, behaviorism, and humanistic psychology. Positive psychology began as a domain of psychology in 1998 when Martin Seligman chose it as the theme for his term as president of the American Psychological Association. Unlike past psychology practices, which empha-sized maladaptive behaviors and negative thinking, positive psychology emphasizes human strengths that promote authentic happiness. Many of the strengths identified were portrayed centuries ago in the Bible, such as love, kindness, forgiveness, self-control, humility, gratitude, integrity, humor, creativity, purpose, excellence, prudence, leadership, fairness, teamwork, and perseverance. Additional positive traits identified included social intelligence, curiosity, appreciation of beauty, optimism, perspective, love of learning, open-mindedness, bravery, and enthusiasm. Preliminary studies are encour-aging among those given assignments based on positive strengths compared to placebo participants. Proponents of positive psychology hope to see more therapists incorporate these interventions. [5]

Your spiritual beliefs play an essential role in your emotional health. Having a connection with your Creator can be a great source of comfort, strength, hope, and healing.

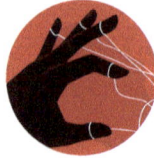

Selah

PAUSE AND THINK ABOUT IT

One of my primary goals in writing this book is to create a paradigm shift from old beliefs about emotional health to empowering beliefs that can reignite your intuition that may have been silenced over time.

Here are some ways you can do this:

- Nurture healthy relationships and ask for support when needed.
- Incorporate movement, sunshine, and gratitude into your day.
- Nourish your body with foods that promote longevity and emotional health.
- Reduce the toxic load on your body and mind.
- Forgive quickly and completely. Refuse to align with negativity.
- Make room for community, creativity, celebration, and fun.
- Find some comic relief. Laughter is good medicine for the body and the soul.
- Connect with your Creator daily to receive wisdom and revelation. God's truth will set you free and give lasting peace to your soul.

My hope is for you to become the unique expression of your Creator that he intended for you to be. By uncovering and untangling emotional chaos, you will be free to achieve all you were designed to be. Let's continue the dialogue. I would love to hear from you.

For the latest information and free resources, subscribe to my email list at *WholisticTransformation.net*. You will be the first to get updates and access to free webinars. You can also request to schedule a seminar online or in person.

Wishing you peace, health, and vitality!

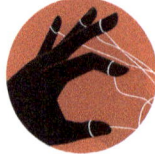

ACKNOWLEDGEMENTS

WITH GRATITUDE . . .

I am eternally grateful for the incredible support I have received along my journey as a first-time author. Those listed here are the most outstanding, although there are countless others that have encouraged me, provided feedback, and nudged me to step out of my comfort zone to document and share what I have learned.

To my mother, who overcame great adversity with dignity and grace. You remained strong in your faith through it all, ensuring your children felt loved and could rise above earthly challenges with their own faith.

To my father, who chose me as his daughter and changed the trajectory of an insecure, directionless, 13-year-old with a strong will. Your life is an expression of the love of our Heavenly Father.

Thank you both for your unconditional love and support that has encouraged me in all my endeavors, even when that path took me far from home.

To my sister Elaine, my first eternal friend who introduced me to the world of health and nutrition. You are a living example of unconditional love and loyalty, supporting me in all seasons of my life. Your faith elevates mine.

To my brother David, the best brother and one of my favorite people in the world. You are always there when I need you, even when it meant learning how to build an herb press for my formulas. Your positive energy and sense of humor are gifts to me and the world.

To my cousin Donna Peake, my soul sister who has traveled this earthly path with me in all ways from the beginning. Your love and support have been a tower of strength for me throughout my life.

To Janet Shaver, my forever friend and faithful prayer warrior. I always feel loved and encouraged in your presence. God smiled when we became friends.

To my friend and mentor, Mary Lee Mahon, for introducing me to the teachings of Dr. R. John Christopher and herbalism. You unlocked a hidden treasure in me.

To my many spiritual sisters for believing in me, laughing with me, and encouraging me when I didn't have the time or motivation to keep writing. Though space does not permit me to mention each of you personally, you know who you are.

To Dr. Lynn Hiles for your solid biblical teaching that has revealed the heart of God to me in a profound way that has deeply impacted my life as a believer.

To Dr. Ed Smith and Joshua Smith for the ongoing training in Transformation Prayer Ministry that continues to transform my life and those I mentor.

To David Christopher and (the late) Dr. R. John Christopher for your wisdom and education that have grounded me on the herbalism path.

To the many brothers and sisters who have bravely gone through the spiritual, emotional, and physical transformation process, allowing me to be part of that sacred journey. You are my heroes for eternity.

I love you all to heaven and back!

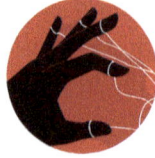

REFERENCES

Chapter 1

ENDNOTES

Physiological Contributors

1. David S. Goldstein and Bruce McEwen, "Allostasis, Homeostats, and the Nature of Stress," *The International Journal on the Biology of Stress,* 5(1) (2009), 55–58, https://doi.org/10.1080/102538902900012345

2. Sara Gottfried, *The Hormone Cure: Reclaim Balance, Sleep and Sex Drive; Lose Weight; Feel Focused, Vital, and Energized Naturally with the Gottfried Protocol* (Scribner, a Division of Simon & Schuster, Inc., 2013), 114.

3. Trudy Scott, "Natural Solutions for Anxiety," *The Anxiety Summit.* https://season2.theanxietysummit.com

4. Sung Ho Maeng and Heeok Hong, "Inflammation As the Potential Basis In Depression," *International Neurourology Journal* (Suppl 2): S63–71 (2019), 113, https://www.ncbi.nlm.nih.gov/pmc/articles/PMC6905209/

5. Debra Umberson and Jennifer Karas Montez, "Social Relationships and Health: A Flashpoint for Health Policy," *Journal of Health and Social Behavior,* 51(1), (2010) S54–S66, https://doi.org/10.1177/0022146510383501

6. "Harlow's Monkey Experiment—The Bond Between Babies and Mothers," *The Psychology Notes HQ* (2020), https://www.psychologynoteshq.com/harlows-monkey-experiment/

7. Eric R. Braverman, *Younger Brain, Sharper Mind: A 6-Step Plan for Preserving and Improving Memory and Attention at Any Age from America's Brain Doctor* (Rodale Books, 2013), 5.

8. Hyla Cass and Patrick Holford, *Natural Highs: Supplements, Nutrition, and Mind-Body Techniques to Help You Feel Good All the Time* (Penguin-Putman Avery Trade, NY, 2003), 114.

9. Michelle Pugle, "What Are Endorphins?" *Verywell Health* (July 26, 2021), https://www.verywellhealth.com/endorphins-definition-5189854

10. Braverman, *Younger Brain, Sharper Mind*, 6.

Environmental Contributors

11. "Body Burden: The Pollution in Newborns," *Environmental Working Group (EWG)*, (July 14, 2005), https://www.ewg.org/research/body-burden-pollution-new-borns

12. Anthony Samsel and Stephanie Seneff, "Glyphosate, Pathways to Modern Diseases II: Celiac Sprue and Gluten Intolerance," *Interdisciplinary Toxicology: Sciendo* 6(4) (2013): 159–184, https://doi.org/10.2478/intox-2013-0026

13. Russell L. Blaylock, *Health and Nutrition Secrets That Can Save Your Life: Harness Your Body's Natural Healing Powers* (Health Press, 2006), 205.

14. Michael T. Dinwiddie, Paul D. Terry, and Jiangang Chen, "Recent Evidence Regarding Triclosan and Cancer Risk," *International Journal of Environmental Research and Public Health*, 11(2) (2014) 2209–2217, https://doi.org/10.3390/ijerph110202209

15. Blaylock, *Health and Nutrition*, 40, 44–45.

16. Blaylock, *Health and Nutrition*, 42, 45, 47.

17. L. Tomljenovic and C. A. Shaw, "Aluminum Vaccine Adjuvants: Are They Safe?" *Current Medicinal Chemistry*, 18(17) (2011), 2630–2637, https://doi.org/10.2174/092986711795933740

18. Wendy Myers, "4 Hidden Sources of Aluminum," Myers Detox™, https://myersdetox.com/4-hidden-sources-of-aluminum/

19. Centers for Disease Control and Prevention (CDC), *Adjuvants*, https://www.cdc.gov/vaccinesafety/concerns/adjuvants.html#

20. Global Skywatch, "What is Geoengineering ("Chemtrails")?" (2010), http://globalskywatch.com/what-are-chemtrails.html

21. Russell L. Blaylock, "What Chemtrails Are Doing to Your Brain—Neurosurgeon Dr. Russell Blaylock Reveals Shocking Facts," *Educate Yourself: The Freedom*

of Knowledge, The Power of Thought (September 2, 2013), http://educate-yourself.org/cn/blaylockchemtraildamagebrain02sep13.shtml

22. K. Buchner K and H. Eger, "Modification of clinically important neurotransmitters under the influence of modulated high-frequency fields—A long-term study under true-to-life conditions," *EMF-Portal* (2011), https://www.emf-portal.org/en/article/19075

23. Gary Gonzalez, "The Hidden Dangers of Cell Phone Radiation, *Life Extension Manazine* (reiewed August 2023), https://www.lifeextension.com/magazine/2007/8/report_cellphone_radiation

24. Nick Pineault, "How 5G and EMF Radiation Impact Your Health," MindBody Medicine Center (2021), https://www.healmindbody.com/how-5g-emf-radiation-impact-your-health/

25. Peter Elkind, "What to Know About Cellphone Radiation," *ProPublica* (January 4), https://www.propublica.org/article/what-to-know-about-cellphone-radiation

26. Martin L. Pall, "Electromagnetic fields act via activation of voltage-gated calcium channels to produce beneficial or adverse effects," *Journal of Cellular and Molecular Medicine*, 17(8) (2013) 958–965, https://www.emfanalysis.com/wp-content/uploads/2015/06/EMF-Effects-via-Voltage-Gated-Calcium-Channels-Dr-Martin-Pall.pdf

27. Dominique Belpomme, Lenmart Hardell, Igor Belyaev, Ernesto Burgio, and David O. Carpenter, "Thermal and non-thermal health effects of low intensity non-ionizing radiation: An international perspective," *Environmental Pollution,* (November 2018) 242 (Part A) 643–658, https://doi.org/10.1016/j.envpol.2018.07.019

28. Lenmart Hardell and Michael Carlberg "Using the Hill viewpoints from 1965 for evaluating strengths of evidence of the risk for brain tumors associated with use of mobile and cordless phones," *Reviews On Environmental Health* (De Gruyter: 2013) 28(2-3), 97–106, https://doi.org/10.1515/reveh-2013-0006

29. BioInnitiative 2012, "BioInitiative Report: Medical concerns intensify over deadly brain tumors from cell phone use" (Orebro University Hospital, Sweden: 2017). http://www.bioinitiative.org/bioinitiative-report-medical-concerns-intensify-over-deadly-brain-tumors-from-cell-phone-use-orebro-university-hospital-sweden-november-17-2017/

30. Cindy Sage and Ernesto Burgio, "Electromagnetic Fields, Pulsed Radiofrequency Radiation, and Epigenetics: How Wireless Technologies May Affect Childhood Development," *Child Development,* 89(1) (Society of Research in Child Development: 2017) 129–135. https://srcd.onlinelibrary.wiley.com/doi/abs/10.1111/cdev.12824

31. Sandro La Vignera, Rosita A. Condorelli, Enzo Vicari, Rosario D'Agata, and Aldo E. Calogero, "Effects of the Exposure to Mobile Phones On Male Reproduction: A Review of the Literature," *Journal of Andrology*, 33(3) (2013) 350–356, https://doi.org/10.2164/jandrol.111.014373

32. Conrado Avendaño, Ariela Mata, Sanchez, César A. Sarmiento, and Gustavo F. Doncel, "Use of laptop computers connected to internet through Wi-Fi decreases human sperm motility and increases sperm DNA fragmentation," *Fertility and Sterility*, 97(1), (January 2012) 39–45 E2, https://doi.org/10.1016/j.fertnstert.2011.10.012

33. Joseph Mercola, "Why Blue Light Is 'Toxic' to Your Eyes," *Mercola: Take Control of Your Health* (August 12, 2018), https://blogs.mercola.com/sites/vitalvotes/archive/2018/08/12/why-blue-light-is-toxic-to-your-eyes.aspx

34. Jospeh Mercola, "LED Light's Health Dangers Confirmed—Don't Be In the Dark!" *Mercola: Take Control of Your Health* (May 24, 2019), https://blogs.mercola.com/sites/vitalvotes/archive/2019/05/24/led-lights-health-dangers-confirmed-dont-be-in-the-dark.aspx

35. PMHNPEXAM, "The Surprising Way Blue Light Impacts Mental and Physical Health," (October 20, 2018), https://pmhnpexam.com/the-surprising-way-blue-light-impacts-mental-and-physical-health/

36. Harvard Medical School, "Blue light has a dark side," (Harvard Health Publishing: July 7, 2020), https://www.health.harvard.edu/staying-healthy/blue-light-has-a-dark-side

37. Blue Light Exposed, "What is blue light?" http://www.bluelightexposed.com/#what-is-blue-light

38. Judy Tsafrir, M.D., "Toxic Mold and Psychiatric Symptoms," (December 13, 2016), https://www.judytsafrirmd.com/toxic-mold-and-psychiatric-symptoms/

39. Chris Kresser, "7 Ways Toxic Mold Affects Your Brain" (June 5, 2020) (originally published by *Paleo Magazine*), https://chriskresser.com/7-ways-toxic-mold-affects-your-brain

40. Amy Myers, "Mycotoxin Poisoning & Toxic Mold: Symptoms & Solutions," (November 10, 2021), https://www.amymyersmd.com/article/toxic-mod/

41. Edward D. Shenassa, Constantine Daskalakis, Allison Liebhaber, Matthias Braubach, and MaryJean Brown, "Dampness and Mold In the Home and Depression: an Examination of Mold-Related Illness and Perceived Control of One's Home as Possible Depression Pathways," *American Journal of Public Health* 97(10) (2007): 1893–1899, https://doi.org/10.2105/AJPH.2006.093773

42. Shenassa, "Dampness and Mold."

43. L. D. Empting, "Neurologic and neuropsychiatric syndrome features of mold and mycotoxin exposure," *Sage Journals: Toxicology and Industrial Health* 25(9-10) (2009), 577–581.8, https://doi.org/10.1177/0748233709348393

44. Tsafrir, "Toxic Mold."

45. Kresser "7 Ways."

46. Myers, "Mycotoxin Poisoning."

47. International Society for Environmentally Acquired Illness (ISEAI), *About ISEAI—Environmentally Acquired Illness*, https://iseai.org/about-eai/

Pharmaceutical Contributors

48. David Perlmutter, "Your Brain Needs Cholesterol" (November 14, 2013), https://www.drperlmutter.com/brain-needs-cholesterol/

49. Stephanie Seneff, "APOE-4: The Clue to Why Low-Fat Diet and Statins May Cause Alzheimer's," (Massachusetts Institute of Technology (MIT): December 15, 2009), http://people.csail.mit.edu/seneff/alzheimers_statins.html

50. Rebecca West, Michal Schnaider Beeri, James Schmeidler, Hillel Grossman, Clive Rosendorff, and Jeremy Silverman, "Better Memory Functioning Is Associated With Higher Total and Low-Density Lipoprotein Cholesterol Levels In Very Elderly Subjects without the Apolipoprotein e4 Allele," *The American Journal of Geriatric Psychiatry*, 16(9) (2008) 781–785, https://doi.org/10.1097/JGP.obo13e3181812790

51. Marcella A. Evans and Beatrice A. Golomb, "Statin-Associated Adverse Cognitive Effects: Survey Results from 171 Patients," *Pharmacotherapy: The Journal of Human Pharmacology and Drug Therapy*, 29(7) (06 January 2009) 800–811, https://doi.org/10.1592/phco.29.7.800

52. Kelly Brogan and Kristin Loberg, *A Mind of Your Own: The Truth About Depression and How Women Can Heal Their Bodies to Reclaim Their Lives* (New York, NY: HarperCollins, 2016), Kindle edition, 2–5.

53. Helen Fisher, "Why we love, why we cheat," *TED*2006, https://www.ted.com/talks/helen_fisher_why_we_love_why_we_cheat

54. Neil Risch, Richard Herrell, Thomas Lehner, Kung-Yee Liang, Lindon Eaves, Josephine Hoh, Andrea Griem, Maria Kovacs, Jung Ott, and Kathleen Ries Merikangas, "Interaction Between the Serotonin Transporter Gene (5-HTTLPR), Stressful Life Events, and Risk of Depression: A Meta-analysis," *JAMA 2009*; 301(23):

2462–2471, https://jamanetwork.com/journals/jama/article-abstract/184107?resultClick=1

55. Paul W. Andrews, Aadil Bharwani, Kyuwon R. Lee, Molly Fox, and J. Anderson Thomson Jr., "Is serotonin an upper or a downer? The evolution of the serotonergic system and its role in depression and the antidepressant response," *Neuroscience & Biobehavioral Reviews*, Vol. 51, April 2015, 164-188, https://doi.org/10.1016/j.neubiorev.2015.01.018

56. Peter Simons, "Researcher Challenges Clinical Effectiveness of Antidepressants," *Mad in America* (September 11, 2018), https://www.madinamerica.com/2018/09/hengartner_clinical_efficacy_adm/

57. Jonathan Price, Victoria Cole, and Guy M. Goodwin, "Emotional side-effects of selective serotonin reuptake inhibitors: qualitative study," *The British Journal of Psychiatry* 195(3) (Cambridge University Press: 2018) 211-217, https://doi.org/10.1192/bjp.bp.108.051110

58. Nassima Ait-Daoud, Allan Scott Hamby, Sana Sharma, and Derek Blevins, "A Review Of Alprazolam Use, Misuse, and Withdrawal," *Journal of Addiction Medicine*, 12(1) (2018) 4–10, https://doi.org/10.1097/ADM.0000000000000350

59. Tobin T. George and Jayson Tripp, "Alprazolam," (StatPearls Publishing: January 2023), www.ncbi.nlm.nih.gov/books/NBK538165/

60. Drugs.com, "Xanax side effects" (September 26, 2002), https://www.drugs.com/sfx/xanax-side-effects.html

61. Suzy Cohen, *Drug Muggers: Which Medications Are Robbing Your Body Essential Nutrients—and Natural Ways to Restore Them* (Rodale: 2011) 108, 203.

62. Lisa Bloomquist, "The Fluoroquinolone Time Bomb — Answers in the Mitochondria," *Hormones Matter* (June 29, 2017), http://www.hormonesmatter.com/fluoroquinolone-time-bomb-mitochondria-damage/

63. MTHFR Living, "Did I get floxed?" (April 11, 2014), http://mthfrliving.com/health-conditions/fluoroquinolones-floxed/

64. Krzysztof Michalak, Aleksandra Sobolewska-Włodarczyk, Marcin Włodarczyk, Justyna Sobolewska, Piotr Woźniak, and Bogusław Sobolewski, "Treatment of the Fluoroquinolone-Associated Disability: The Pathobiochemical Implications," *Oxidative Medicine And Cellular Longevity*, Vol. 2017, Article ID 8023935 (29 Sept 2017), https://doi.org/10.1155/2017/8023935

65. Neil Paulvin, "Fluoroquinolone Toxicity Symptoms from a Functional Medicine Perspective," *What to Do When You Get Floxed: Recovery & Healing from Fluoroquinolone Toxicity*, (April 17, 2021), https://doctorpaulvin.com/blog/what-to-do-when-you-get-floxed/

66. U.S. Food and Drug Administration, "FDA Updates Warnings for Fluoroquinolone Antibiotics," (July 26, 2016), https://www.fda.gov/news-events/press-announcements/fda-updates-warnings-fluoroquinolone-antibiotics

67. "Fluoroquinolone Toxicity Psychosis and Depression" (September 27, 2022: Blog 4), Floxie Hope, https://floxiehope.com/fluoroquinolone-toxicity-psychosis-and-depression/

Chapter 2
ENDNOTES

1. Shih-Hsien Lin, Lan-Ting Lee, and Yen Kuang Yang, "Serotonin and Mental Disorders: A Concise Review On Molecular Neuroimaging Evidence," *Clinical Psychopharmacology and Neuroscience,* 12(3) (The Korean College of Neuropsychopharmacology, 2014), 196–202, https://doi.org/10.9758/cpn.2014.12.3.196

2. Philip Strandwitz, "Neurotransmitter modulation by the gut microbiota," *Brain Research,* 1693/Part B (August 2018), 128–133, https://doi.org/10.1016/j.brainres.2018.03.015

3. Amy Myers, M.D., "Serotonin & The Gut: The Gut-Brain Axis," https://www.amymyersmd.com/article/serotonin-gut-health/

4. David Perlmutter and Kristin Loberg, *Grain Brain: The Surprising Truth about Wheat, Carbs, and Sugar—Your Brain's Silent Killer* (New York, NY: Little, Brown Spark, 2013), 51–52, 149, 166–168.

5. Jessica R. Jackson, William W. Eaton, Nicola G. Cascella, Alessio Fasano, and Deanna L. Kelly, "Neurologic And Psychiatric Manifestations Of Celiac Disease And Gluten Sensitivity," *The Psychiatric Quarterly* 83 (2012), 91–102, https://doi.org/10.1007/s11126-011-9186-y

6. Anthony Samsel and Stephanie Seneff, "Glyphosate, pathways to modern diseases II: Celiac sprue and gluten intolerance," *Interdisciplinary Toxicology,* 6(4) (December 2013), 159–184, https://doi.org/10.2478/intox-2013-0026

7. Stephanie Seneff and Ashley James, "259: Glyphosate," *Learn True Health,* https://www.learntruehealth.com/glyphosate

8. Russell L. Blaylock, *Health and Nutrition Secrets That Can Save Your Life: Harness Your Body's Natural Healing Powers* (Albuquerque, NM: Health Press, 2006), 315

9. Andrew Weil, "Can Carbs Cause Alzheimer's?" *Weil,* (May 3, 2013), https://www.drweil.com/health-wellness/health-centers/aging gracefully/can-carbs-cause-alzheimers/

10. M. Regina Castro, "Diabetes and depression: Coping with the two conditions," *Mayo Clinic,* https://www.mayoclinic.org/diseases-conditions/diabetes/expert-answers/diabetes-and-depression/faq-20057904

11. Blaylock, *Health and Nutrition,* 172, 174

12. Peg Desrochers, "Sugar and Gut Health—A Disturbing Connection," *True Gut Health*, https://trueguthealth.com/sugar-and-gut-health/

13. Joseph Mercola, "The Truth about Sugar Addiction," (June 16 2019), *Conscious Life News*, https://consciouslifenews.com/the-truth-about-sugar-addiction-dr-mercola/11170677/

14. Nancy Appleton and G. N. Jacob, *Suicide by Sugar* (Garden City Park, NY: Square One Publishers, 2009), 94-95.

15. B. J. Venn and T. J. Green, "Glycemic Index and Glycemic Load: Measurement Issues and Their Effect on Diet-disease Relationships," *European Journal of Clinical Nutrition*, 61 Suppl 1 (2007): S122–S131, https://doi.org/10.1038/sj.ejcn.1602942

16. Glycemic Index Foundation (n.d.), "Low GI Explained," https://www.gisymbol.com/low-gi-explained/

17. Blaylock, *Health and Nutrition*, 196.

18. Mohamed B. Abou-Donia, Eman M. El-Masry, Ali A. Abdel-Rahman, Roger E. McLendon, and Susan S. Schiffman, "Splenda Alters Gut Microflora and Increases Intestinal P-Glycoprotein and Cytochrome P-450 in Male Rats, *Journal of Toxicology and Environmental Health, Part A*, 71(21) (2008): 1415–1429, https://doi.org/10.1080/15287390802328630

19. Environmental Working Group (EWG), *EWG's Consumer Guide to Seafood* (September 18, 2014), https://www.ewg.org/consumer-guides/ewgs-consumer-guide-seafood

20. Nevin Sanlier, Busra Basar Gökcen, and Aybuke Ceyhun Sezgin, "Health Benefits of Fermented Foods," *Critical Reviews in Food Science and Nutrition*, 59(3), (2019) 506–527, https://doi.org/10.1080/10408398.2017.1383355

21. Roghayeh Shahbazi, Farzaneh Sharifzad, Rana Bagheri, Nawal Alsadil, Hamed Yasavoli-Sharahi, and Chantal Matar, "Anti-inflammatory and Immunomodulatory Properties of Fermented Plant Foods," *Nutrients*, 13(5) (2021): 1516, https://doi.org/10.3390/nu13051516

22. Noriaki Nagai, Yoshimasa Ito, and Atsushi Taga, "Comparison of the Enhancement of Plasma Glucose Levels in Type 2 Diabetes Otsuka Long-Evans Tokushima Fatty Rats by Oral Administration of Sucrose or Maple Syrup," *Journal of Oleo Science*, 62(9) (2013): 737–743, https://doi.org/10.5650/jos.62.737

23. Jean Legault, Karl Girard-Lalancette, Carole Grenon, Catherine Dussault, and Andre Pichette, "Antioxidant Activity, Inhibition of Nitric Oxide Overproduction, and In Vitro Antiproliferative Effect of Maple Sap and Syrup from Acer

Saccharum," *Journal of Medicinal Food*, 13(2) (2010): 460–468, https://doi.org/10.1089/jmf.2009.0029

24. Ty Bollinger, "Fluoride — Drinking Ourselves to Death?," *The Truth About Cancer* (April 12, 2021), https://thetruthaboutcancer.com/fluoride-drinking-ourselves-to-death/

25. Sara Gottfried, *The Hormone Cure* (New York, NY: Scribner, 2013), Kindle edition, 135.

26. Angela Sanford, "Brain Benefits of L-theanine," *Life Extension Magazine*, (March 1, 2016), https://www.lifeextension.com/magazine/2016/3/brain-benefits-of-l-theanine.

27. Nan Hu, Jin-Tai Yu, Lin Tan, Ying-Li Wang, Lei Sun, and Lan Tan, "Nutrition and the Risk of Alzheimer's Disease," *BioMed Research International*, Vol. 2013, Article ID 524820 (2013): 12 pages, https://doi.org/10.1155/2013/524820

28. Kenta Kimura, Makoto Ozeki, Lekh Raj Juneja, and Hideki Ohirai, "L-Theanine Reduces Psychological and Physiological Stress Responses," *Biological Psychology*, 74(1) (2007): 39–45, https://doi.org/10.1016/j.biopsycho.2006.06.00

29. David Perlmutter and Kristin Loberg, *Brain Maker: The Power of Gut Microbes to Heal and Protect Your Brain for Life* (New York, NY: Little, Brown and Company, 2015), 51–52, 60–62.

Chapter 3

ENDNOTES

1. Mark Hyman, "Here's How to Heal Our Broken Brains With Nutrients," *Broken Brains*, https://drhyman.com/blog/2018/01/16/heres-heal-broken-brains-nutrients/

2. Russell L. Blaylock, *Health and Nutrition Secrets That Can Save Your Life: Harness Your Body's Natural Healing Powers* (Health Press, 2006), 152, 323.

3. Blaylock, *Health and Nutrition Secrets,* 322.

4. Blaylock, *Health and Nutrition Secrets,* 322.

5. Kelly Brogan and Kristin Loberg, *A Mind of Your Own: The Truth about Depression and How Women Can Heal Their Bodies to Reclaim Their Lives* (New York, NY: HarperCollins, 2016), Kindle edition, 224–225

6. Margaret E. Sears, "Chelation: Harnessing and Enhancing Heavy Metal Detoxification—A Review," *The Scientific World Journal*, Vol. 2013, Article ID 219840 (2013): 13 pages, https://doi.org/10.1155/2013/219840

7. Blaylock, *Health and Nutrition Secrets,* 322.

8. Brisa S. Fernandes, Olivia M. Dean, Seetal Dodd, Gin A. Malhi, and Michael Berk, "N-Acetylcysteine in Depressive Symptoms and Functionality: A Systematic Review and Meta-analysis," *The Journal of Clinical Psychiatry,* 77(4) (2016): e457–e466, https://doi.org/10.4088/JCP.15r09984

9. K. Paydary, A. Akamaloo, A. Ahmadipour, F. Pishgar, S. Emamzadehfard, and S. Akhondzadeh, "N-acetylcysteine Augmentation Therapy for Moderate-to-Severe Obsessive-Compulsive Disorder: Randomized, Double-Blind, Placebo-Controlled Trial," *Journal of Clinical Pharmacy and Therapeutics,* 41(2) (2016): 214–219, https://doi.org/10.1111/jcpt.12370

10. B. Pósfai, C. Cserép, P. Hegedüs, E. Szabadits, D. M. Otte, A. Zimmer, M. Watanabe, T. F. Freund, and G. Nyiri, "Synaptic and Cellular Changes Induced by the Schizophrenia Susceptibility Gene G72 are Rescued by N-acetylcysteine Treatment," *Translational Psychiatry,* 6(5) (2016): e807, https://doi.org/10.1038/tp.2016.74

Chapter 4

ENDNOTES

1. Barbara Griggs, *Green Pharmacy (3rd ed)* (Healing Arts Press, 1997), 1.

2. Russell L. Blaylock, *Health and Nutrition Secrets That Can Save Your Life: Harness Your Body's Natural Healing Powers* (Health Press, 2006), 321.

3. John R. Christopher, *Herb Syllabus* (Springville, UT: Christopher Publications, 2010), 244.

4. Alan Keith Tillotson, Nai-shing Hu Tillotson, and Robert Abel Jr., *The One Earth Herbal Sourcebook* (New York, NY: Kensington Publishing, 2001), 138, 139.

5. Pierre L. Le Bars, Martin M. Katz, Nancy Berman, Turan M. Itil, Alfred M. Freedman, and Alan F. Schatzberg, "A Placebo-Controlled, Double-blind, Randomized Trial of an Extract of Ginkgo Biloba for Dementia," *JAMA*, 278(16) (1997): 1327–1332, https://jamanetwork.com/journals/jama/article-abstract/418442

6. American Botanical Council, "Ginkgo Biloba Leaf Extract," (July 19, 1994), https://www.herbalgram.org/resources/commission-e-monographs/approved-herbs/ginkgo-biloba-leaf-extract/

7. Amanda Chan, "Rosemary Brain Benefit: Study Shows Link Between Herb Chemical and Brainpower," *Huffpost* (February 27, 2012), https://www.huffpost.com/entry/rosemary-brain-memory-18-cineole_n_1304250

8. Natasha K. Wolfe, Douglas I. Katz, Matthew L. Albert, Avraham Almozlino, Rosaria D'Urso, Miranda Caroline Smith, and Ladislav Volicer, "Neuropsychological Profile Linked to Low Dopamine: in Alzheimer's Disease, Major Depression, and Parkinson's Disease," *Journal of Neurology, Neurosurgery and Psychiatry*, 53(10) (1990): 915–917, https://www.ncbi.nlm.nih.gov/pmc/articles/PMC488258/

9. Mark Moss and Lorraine Oliver, "Plasma 1,8-cineole Correlates with Cognitive Performance Following Exposure to Rosemary Essential Oil Aroma," *Therapeutic Advances in Psychopharmacology*, Vol. 2,3 (2012): 103–13, https://doi.org/10.1177/2045125312436573

10. Mark Moss, Jenny Cook, Keith Wesnes, and Paul Duckett, "Aromas of Rosemary and Lavender Essential Oils Differentially Affect Cognition and Mood in Healthy Adults," *International Journal of Neuroscience*, 113 (2003): 15–38, https://pubmed.ncbi.nlm.nih.gov/12690999/

11. National Institutes of Health, "Valerian: Fact Sheet for Health Professionals," (March 15, 2013), http://ods.od.nih.gov/factsheets/Valerian-Health-Professional/

12. Margaret Grieve, *A Modern Herbal: The Medicinal, Culinary, Cosmetic and Economic Properties, Cultivation and Folk-Lore of Herbs, Grasses, Fungi, Shrubs, and Trees with Their Modern Scientific Uses* (New York, NY: Hafner Press, 1974), 824–830.

13. Nicholas Culpeper, *Culpeper's Complete Herbal: Over 400 Herbs and Their Uses* (New York, NY: W. Foulsham, 1994), 295–297.

14. Christopher, *Herb Syllabus*, 665.

15. Tara Bassi, "American Skullcap: 5 Key Benefits, Dosage, and Safety," *The Botanical Institute*, (February 3, 2022), https://botanicalinstitute.org/american-skullcap/

16. Christopher, *Herb Syllabus*, 36, 38

17. James J. Duke, *The Green Pharmacy: The Ultimate Compendium Of Natural Remedies From The World's Foremost Authority On Healing Herbs* (New York, NY: St. Martin's Paperbacks, 1997), 157–158.

18. Jintaporn Wattanathorn, Lugkana Mator, Supaporn Muchimapura, Terdthai Tongun, Orapin Pasuriwong, Nawanant Piyawatkul, Kwanchanok Yimtae, Bungorn Sripanidkulchai, and Jintana Singkhoraard, "Positive Modulation of Cognition and Mood in the Healthy Elderly Volunteer Following the Administration of Centella Asiatica," *Journal of Ethnopharmacology*, 116(2) (2008): 325–332, https://doi.org/10.1016/j.jep.2007.11.038

19. Chris Kilham, "Peruvian Power Plant," *Medicine Hunter*, (2008), https://www.medicinehunter.com/peruvian-power-plant

20. Christopher Hobbs, "Herbal Adaptogens Fitting Into the Modern Age," *Healthy*, https://healthy.net/2000/12/06/herbal-adaptogens-fitting-into-the-modern-age/?cn-reloaded=1

21. Adaptongens.org, "The Orchestration of a Dream," (2021), http://www.adaptogens.org/research/brekhman/brekhman.html

22. Chris Kilham, "Eluthrococcus," *Adaptongens.org* (2021), http://www.adaptogens.org/plants/Eleutherococcus.html

23. Chris Kilham, "Rhodiola Rosea," *Medicine Hunter*, (2010), http://www.medicinehunter.com/rhodiola

24. Sara Gottfried, *The Hormone Cure* (New York, NY: Scribner, 2013), Kindle edition, 143

25. Alesander Bystritsky, Lauren Kerwin, and Jamie D. Feusner, "A Pilot Study of Rhodiola Rosea (Rhodax) for Generalized Anxiety Disorder (GAD)," *Journal of Alternative and Complementary Medicine* 14(2) (2008): 175–180, https://doi.org/10.1089/acm.2007.7117

26. Dnyanraj Choudhary, Sauvik K. Bhattacharyya, and Sekhar Bose, "Efficacy and Safety of Ashwagandha (Withania somnifera (L.) Dunal) Root Extract in Improving Memory and Cognitive Functions." *Journal of Dietary Supplements* Vol. 14,6 (2017): 599–612, https://doi.org/10.1080/19390211.2017.1284970

27. Sauvik K. Bhattacharya, Arunabh Bhattacharya, Sairam Krishnamurthy, and Sriparna Ghosal, "Anxiolytic-antidepressant Activity of Withania Somnifera Glycowithanolides: An Experimental Study," *Phytomedicine: International Journal of Phytotherapy and Phytopharmacology*, 7(6) (2000): 463–469, https://doi.org/10.1016/S0944-7113(00)80030-6

28. Chris Kilham, "Maca and the Medicine Hunter," *Medicine Hunter*, http://www.medicinehunter.com/maca

29. Jie Li, Jian Wang, Jia-qing Shao, Hong Du, Yang-tian Wang, and Li Peng, "Effect of Schisandra Chinensis on Interleukins, Glucose Metabolism, and Pituitary-adrenal and Gonadal Axis in Rats Under Strenuous Swimming Exercise." *Chinese Journal of Integrative Medicine*, 21(1) (2015): 43–48, https://doi.org/10.1007/s11655-014-1765-y

30. Ling-Jun Sun, Guo-Hong Wang, Bo Wu, Jian Wang, Qun Wang, Lan Ping Hu, Jia-QingShao, Yang-Tian Wang, Jie Li, Ping Gu, and Bin Lu, "Effects of Schisandra on the Function of the Pituitary-Adrenal Cortex, Gonadal Axis and Carbohydrate Metabolism in Rats Undergoing Experimental Chronic Psychological Stress, Navigation and Strenuous Exercise," *Zhonghua Nan Ke Xue*, 15(2) (2009): 126–129, https://pubmed.ncbi.nlm.nih.gov/19323371/

Chapter 5

ENDNOTES

1. Thomas DeLauer, "Most People Do HIIT Cardio Wrong—How to Do HIIT," March 16, 2018, 5:28 min., https://youtu.be/5O1TTduK6mw

2. Brett R. Gordon, Cillian P. McDowell, Mats Hallgren, Jacob D. Meyer, Mark Lyons, and Matthew P. Herring, "Association of Efficacy of Resistance Exercise Training With Depressive Symptoms: Meta-analysis and Meta-regression Analysis of Randomized Clinical Trials," *JAMA Psychiatry*, 75(6) (2018): 566–576, https://doi.org/10.1001/jamapsychiatry.2018.0572

3. James L. Oschman, Gaetan Chevalier, and Clinton Ober, "Biophysics of Earthing (Grounding) the Human Body," reprint from *Bioelectromagnetic and Subtle Energy Medicine, 2nd Edition* (New York, NY: CRC Press, 2015), 427–448.

4. Clinton Ober, Stephen T. Sinatra, and Martin Zucker, *Earthing: The Most Important Health Discovery Ever!* (Laguna Beach, CA: Basic Health Publications, Inc., 2010), 61, 103, 145.

5. RTOG Foundation, "Depression, Anxiety, Mental Health and Chiropractic Care," (February 21, 2019), https://www.rtor.org/2019/02/21/mental-health-and-chiropractic-care

6. Mayo Clinic Press, "Mayo Clinic Explores: The role of massage therapy for mental health," (November 2, 2021), https://mcpress.mayoclinic.org/emotional-health/mayo-clinic-explores-the-role-of-massage-therapy-for-mental-health/

7. Nick Ortner, "What is Tapping and How Does It Work?, *The Tapping Solution,* https://www.thetappingsolution.com/blog/what-is-tapping/

8. Norman Cousins, "Anatomy of an Illness as Perceived by the Patient: Reflections on Healing and Regeneration," *Academia,* https://www.academia.edu/35082295/Anatomy_of_an_Illness_As_perceived_by_the_Patient_Reflections_on_Healing_and_Regeneration

9. Michele M. Tugade, Barbara L. Fredrickson, and Lisa Feldman Barrett, "Psychological Resilience and Positive Emotional Granularity: Examining the Benefits of Positive Emotions on Coping and Health," *Journal of Personality* 72(6), 1161–1190 (2004), https://doi.org/10.1111/j.1467-6494.2004.00294.x

10. Mell Johnson, "The Story Behind the Hymn 'It Is Well with My Soul,'" *Inspirational Stories* (March 7, 2016), https://www.godupdates.com/story-behind-it-is-well-with-my-soul/

Chapter 6

ENDNOTES

1. Bruce Lipton, *The Biology of Belief, 10th Anniversary Edition (2nd ed.)* (Carlsbad, CA: Hay House, 2016), 43.

2. Lipton, *The Biology of Belief*, xv.

3. Lipton, *The Biology of Belief*, 122.

4. Lipton, *The Biology of Belief*, 128.

Chapter 7

ENDNOTES

1. Ed Smith and Joshua Smith, *Effortless Forgiveness* (Campbellsville, KY: New Creation Publishing, 2018), 93–95.

2. Frank Meadows, *Understanding Dissociation*. Seminar presented at North Way Christian Community, Wexford, PA (2007, October 27).

Chapter 8

ENDNOTES

1. Ed Smith and Joshua Smith, *Transformation Prayer Ministry* (Simpsonville, SC: New Creation Publishing, 2023), 45.

Chapter 9

ENDNOTES

1. Megan Cerullo, "First Responders More Likely to Die from Suicide Than in Line of Duty," *Daily News* (April 12, 2018), http://www.nydailynews.com/news/national/responders-die-suicide-job-article-1.3930162

Chapter 10

ENDNOTES

1. Bruce Lipton, *The Biology of Belief, 10th Anniversary Edition (2nd ed.)* (Carlsbad, CA: Hay House, 2016), 221.

2. Harold G. Koenig, "Religion, Spirituality, and Health: The Research and Clinical Implications," *International Scholarly Research Notices*, Vol. 2012, Article ID 278730, (2012): 33 pages, https://doi.org/10.5402/2012/278730

3. Stephanie A. Bosco-Ruggiero, "The Relationship Between Americans' Spiritual/Religious Beliefs and Behaviors and Mental Health: New Evidence from the 2016 General Social Survey," *Journal of Spirituality in Mental Health*, 22(1) (2020): 3048, https://doi.org/10.1080/19349637.2018.1515052

4. David R. Brown, Jamie S. Carney, Mark S. Parrish, and John L. Klem, "Assessing Spirituality: The Relationship Between Spirituality and Mental Health," *Journal of Spirituality in Mental Health*, 15(2) (2013): 107–122, https://doi.org/10.1080/19349637.2013.776442

5. Martin Seligman, "The New Era of Positive Psychology," *TED*, https://youtu.be/9FBxfd7DL3E

About the Author

Sandra Casciato is a wholistic wellness consultant and educator with more than 20 years' experience specializing in herbalism and emotional wellness. She received her master of herbology from the School of Natural Healing and has developed five original herbal formulas. As a wellness consultant, she provides individual consultations and group wellness seminars. To learn more, visit *WholisticTransformation.net*.

www.ingramcontent.com/pod-product-compliance
Lightning Source LLC
Chambersburg PA
CBHW070127030426
42335CB00016B/2295

*9 7 9 8 9 8 7 2 6 4 2 0 1 *